INSTRUMENTATION
IN MEDICINE

INSTRUMENTATION IN MEDICINE

Essays by members of the Department of
Chemical Physics and Bio-engineering
Western Regional Hospital Board, Glasgow

Edited by

J. M. A. LENIHAN

M.Sc., Ph.D., C.Eng., M.I.E.E., F.Inst. P., F.R.S.E.

MORGAN-GRAMPIAN
LONDON
1968

© J. M. A. Lenihan

A Control Series Book
General Editor, A. Conway

First published in Great Britain 1968 by
Morgan-Grampian Books Ltd
28, Essex Street
Strand, London, W.C.2

Printed in Great Britain by Richard Clay (The Chaucer Press), Ltd.,
Bungay, Suffolk

LIST OF CONTENTS

CONTRIBUTORS

J. M. A. Lenihan, M.Sc., Ph.D., C.Eng., M.I.I.E.E., F.Inst.P., F.R.S.E.
Regional Physicist. Western Regional Hospital Board

J. McKie, B.Sc.
Deputy Regional Physicist

A. H. Etchells, B.Sc.
Assistant Regional Physicist

F. C. Gillespie, B.Sc., Ph.D.
Principal Physicist

D. L. Thomas, B.Sc., Ph.D., C.Eng., M.I.E.E., A.Inst.P.
Principal Physicist

CHAPTER 1

THE LESSONS OF HISTORY

Science, technology and medicine are the principal forces that have shaped the world of today, dominated as it is by man's persistent and, on the whole, successful efforts to gain knowledge and understanding of the material universe as a means of controlling, exploiting and modifying the environment for the common good. The purpose of this book is to illustrate one aspect of the process by studying the relationship of instrument technology to medicine.

In this exploration it is advisable to steer a middle course between the insistent contemporary clamour for the improvement of medicine by a stiff dose of technology and the indifference of the many doctors who believe that gadgets are interesting but irrelevant. Tradition and innovation are both important in the practice of medicine. The current wave of enthusiasm for technology is perhaps a natural reaction after centuries in which tradition seemed to be dominant. But the patient does not always want to be treated with scientific detachment or technical ingenuity. He is supported by the belief that every disease has a cure, which he confidently expects his medical advisers to produce for him. This belief may be dismissed as merely magical, but it has sustained physicians and their patients down the ages and will not be seriously undermined by any amount of progress in the laboratory or the development workshop.

Though medicine sometimes appears to lean heavily on authority and on long-established knowledge, it is by no means an unadventurous activity. Indeed, the association of science and technology with medicine has been very much closer in the past than it is today. For a long time there were no professional scientists, for the doctor was the only man to receive any scientific education. Systematic teaching of chemistry as a separate discipline did not start until about 200 years ago. Physicists did not arise in appreciable numbers until well into the nineteenth century, and the emergence of the biological sciences is even more recent.

The foundations supporting the contemporary association between science and technology were, in many instances, built by medical men, to whom the practice of science was a natural extension of their clinical efforts. William Gilbert, the first English physicist, was Queen Elizabeth's physician. His work on magnetism contributed significantly to the important technology of navigation and, by suggesting the possibility of action at a distance, paved the way for later work on gravitation. Joseph Black, whose discovery of latent heat provided the scientific basis for the Industrial Revolution, was professor of medicine at Glasgow University. Thomas Young, who established the wave theory of light, edited the Britannica and deciphered the Rosetta Stone, was physician to St George's Hospital in London—and, incidentally, regarded his scientific work as a rather disreputable hobby. Robert Hooke was an honorary Doctor of Medicine (this being the distinction appropriate to an eminent scientist of the seventeenth century). A succession of other great men of science, from Copernicus to Helmholtz, were trained as doctors, and some (including Galileo and Humphry Davy) learned about science while they were medical students, though they never qualified.

It is to the doctors of bygone days that we owe the birth of instrument technology—and, indeed, the basic idea that science can be useful. To the Greek philosophers, the object of studying science (or anything else) was self-improvement; Plato taught that a learned man was also a virtuous man, best fitted to exercise responsibility in the affairs of the state. This principle was not seriously challenged till Paracelsus, the bombastic physician of sixteenth-century Europe, told his fellow-alchemists that they were wasting their time in looking for the philosopher's stone. The true purpose of alchemy, he said, is not to make gold but to find drugs for the relief of suffering. His methods, based on the liberal administration of arsenic, antimony and mercury, were not uniformly successful—but his followers were convinced of the value of the new therapeutics. In the effort to discover why their patients died after the best scientific treatment, they developed the ideas of chemical purity and showed the importance of the quantitative approach, not only in medicine but also in chemistry.

Even before Paracelsus was born, Nicolas of Cusa suggested that measurement has a place in medicine. He proposed the use of the balance in studies of blood and urine, and may also have recommended the counting of the pulse. None of these projects found immediate fulfilment, for the technological means to pursue them were lacking. The time, the man and the machinery did not come together until the early years of the seventeenth century.

The man who founded the practice of instrument technology—and, in a wider sense, established the quantitative approach to medicine—was Sanctorius of Padua, who lived from 1561 to 1636. Educated (like his friend Galileo) in the medical faculty of the University of Padua, he became famous as a physician in Poland and in Venice before returning to his alma mater as professor of medicine in 1611.

His three major contributions to medicine were all distinguished by profound insight as well as technical ingenuity. Sanctorius was the first to measure a patient's pulse rate; what is more important, he was the first to appreciate that a knowledge of the pulse rate would be useful in the diagnosis or management of disease. Until then physicians had studied the quality of the pulse, a property difficult to define but involving the pressure and waveform as estimated by the finger placed over the radial artery.

The technical problem of measuring the pulse rate was formidable, at a time when the stop-watch was unknown and when even the best clocks had only an hour hand. Sanctorius knew of Galileo's discovery (in 1581) that the period of oscillation of a pendulum depended on its length but not on the amplitude of swing. Galileo used the pulse beat as a reference source in this work, and Kepler (1600) used the pulse to indicate the passage of time for astronomical measurements. Sanctorius took a decisive step forward with the invention of the pulsilogium. This was no more than a small lead weight tied to the end of string. The length of the string was adjusted until the swings of the pendulum were synchronous with the pulse beats—an early application of the heterodyne principle.* The pulse rate was noted as a length, allowing comparisons to be made between one day and the next or between one patient and another.

In this achievement, as in much else that he did, Sanctorius was far ahead of his time. The importance of the numerical estimation of pulse rate was hardly recognized during the eighteenth century and did not become a regular part of the physician's examination of the patient until well into the nineteenth century. Even William Harvey (who graduated in Padua in 1602, the year that Sanctorius published his account of the pulsilogium) mentioned the pulse rate only once in all his writings—and observed merely that its rate varied between 1000 and 4000 per half-hour.

The second great invention of Sanctorius was the clinical thermometer. A crude form of thermoscope, in which water or wine was used as the expanding fluid, was known to the Greeks. Sanctorius added a scale to obtain numerical results, and made an instrument with a bulb which could be placed in the mouth. He recognized the value of assessing the degree of heat of the body, even though the notion of temperature was far in the future. His clinical writings in the use of the thermometer are tantalizingly brief, but it seems that he appreciated the value of good temperature records as an aid to the management of fevers. Here again he was ahead of his time, for it was not until nearly 250 years later that thermometry became common in medicine; the modern form of clinical thermometer was invented (by Sir Clifford Allbutt) as recently as 1870. Allbutt, in his zeal to record temperatures in various parts of the body, encountered good-

* I am indebted to J. F. M. Scholes for this comment.

natured opposition from his patients and was offered many ribald comments 'the repetition of which', he wrote drily, 'would not conduce to edification'.

Sanctorius makes a third claim on our attention as the pioneer of metabolic studies, and, it may be asserted without exaggeration, the founder of experimental physiology. His experiments here (described in 'De Statica Medicina', published in 1614) were founded on the recognition of the essential equilibrium underlying the body's ever-changing metabolic processes, based on the exchange and transformation of food and energy. Sanctorius built a steelyard, supporting a cage containing a chair giving access to a table. The system having been initially balanced, changes in the mass of the experimenter, due to ingestion of food, excretion or perspiration, were made evident as vertical displacements of the chair, which could be measured and compensated. His main study was concerned with 'insensible perspiration' as a function of body temperature, sleep or wakefulness, exercise and diet. In these matters the work of Sanctorius was not significantly extended until accurate calorimetry began to be practised towards the end of the eighteenth century.

The ideas of Sanctorius were revolutionary because they were fundamental. It is always easier to make use of existing ideas than to develop new ones. Richard Mead, who was Queen Anne's physician, expressed an acceptable view when he wrote, in 1702, of a novel application for the new ideas advanced by Newton. Doctors, like other wise men of the time, were intrigued by the mechanical explanation of the otherwise supernatural phenomena of gravity and astronomy. A major problem in medicine at that time was the detection and treatment of poisoning. In the preface to 'A Mechanical Account of Poisons' Mead observed: 'My Design in thinking of these Matters was, to try how far I could carry Mechanical Consideration in Accounting for those surprising Changes which Poisons make in an Animal Body. . . .' He did not make much of this endeavour, but the significant point is that he thought it worth while to apply the latest scientific ideas to the attack on an apparently insoluble medical problem. A note of despair (to be echoed by many of his successors) is evident in a later passage: 'It is very evident, that all other Methods of improving Medicine have been found Ineffectual . . . and that since of late Mathematicians have set Themselves to the Study of It, Men do already begin to Talk so Intelligibly and Comprehensibly, even about abstruse Matters, that it may be hoped in a short Time . . . that Mathematical Learning will be the Distinguishing Mark of a Physician from a Quack.' Mead's sentiments, expressed in more up-to-date language, can be heard at the opening of any contemporary symposium on the use of computers in medicine.

Another eighteenth-century novelty was electricity, and the possible applications in medicine received a characteristic assessment from Johann Kruger of Halle in 1743. He told his students that electricity would be important in many ways, though he did not quite see where progress would be concentrated. 'God only knows,' he said, 'what the ingenious heads of our time will get out of it all ... if it must have some practical use, it is certain that none has been found for it in Theology or Jurisprudence, and therefore where else can the use be than in Medicine?'

X-rays, radio-activity, electronics, crystallography, isotopes, computers, solid-state physics, ultrasonics, cryogenics—almost every advance in physical science or the associated technologies has been pressed into the service of medicine, sometimes with spectacular results.

Belief in the virtue of applying the currently fashionable science or technology to difficult problems in medicine is old and respectable. This belief inspires the present-day advocates of interdisciplinary collaboration in medical electronics and biological engineering. It is, to a large extent, a rational and commendable belief, more likely to produce important results today than at any time in the past—not because its exponents are any more able than their forebears down the ages, but simply because the quantity of technology now existing to be plundered is so great that a systematic (or even a random) attack can hardly fail to yield something useful.

The human body is a system of such complexity and subtlety that it can be plausibly described in a great variety of ways. Mead thought that its design and functions were primarily mechancial. At different times it has seemed that convincing explanations might be based on the ideas of chemistry, biochemistry or electronics. In the succeeding chapters we shall not be attempting any speculations of this kind, but shall review the ways in which the practice of instrument technology can help the doctor and the medical research worker. We shall also try to identify some of the areas in which further progress is needed to satisfy the reasonable requirements of the world of medicine.

The body may, as we have seen, be regarded as a chemical works, a telephone exchange or an electronic computer. For our purpose it will be useful to start by looking at its function as a power station, examining the multiplicity of electrical signals generated by various bodily processes and summarizing the information that can be deduced from them. As a complement to this study we shall also look at the possibility of injecting electrical signals to stimulate, augment or replace a deficient natural activity.

There are two main sources of electrical activity in the body— muscle and nerve. Muscular contraction is accompanied by a migration of ions, generating potential differences which can be measured by suitably placed electrodes. The heart, as the most important muscle in the body, has been intensively studied in this way. Even when the electrodes are placed on the wrists, signals of about 1 mV amplitude are recorded. For other muscles it is usually necessary to use needle electrodes, inserted directly into the tissue, when potential differences of up to 100 μV may be detected.

Electrochemical changes associated with the conduction of signals along nerves (to or from the brain) produce potential differences of a few microvolts amplitude. A complicated pattern of electrical activity can be recorded from the brain (even during sleep or rest) by means of electrodes placed on the scalp.

The restoration of palsied muscles by electrical stimuli was one of the first techniques developed as a result of Kruger's encouragement, already mentioned. Kratzenstein and Lange, two of his colleagues in Halle, administered static electricity and claimed remarkable cures. Similar methods are still used, with unsophisticated generators of direct or low-frequency alternating current. More hazardous—but often successful—techniques are available for cardiac pacemaking (when the natural timing mechanism of the heart is out of action) or defibrillation, when a sudden shock will sometimes restore normal rhythmic beating.

These matters (which form the basis of the next chapter) may be investigated with nothing more complicated than electrodes and generating or measuring equipment. In a further range of bodily activities (discussed in chapter 3) information is gathered with the help of transducers applied to external or otherwise accessible locations. Blood pressure and other aspects of the circulation, respiration and lung function, and a variety of problems related to body kinetics, may be studied in this way.

It is often important to learn about the metabolism of particular chemical elements or compounds. Radio-active isotopes have proved immensely useful in this endeavour. In chapter 4 we look at the problems and potentialities of instrumentation associated with isotope techniques, considering both the relatively simple methods for examining uptake, transport, dilution and turnover processes and the more sophisticated recent developments, including whole-body counting and activation analysis.

The fifth chapter is concerned with a group of techniques for delineating various organs of the body and for evaluating their functional performance in health or disease. The oldest major instrument for this purpose, the radiograph, is briefly discussed and attention directed to techniques involving radio-active isotopes (sometimes with scanning display systems), ultrasonics and infra-red radiation.

Chapter 6 covers ground closer to the familiar territory of the instrument technologist, describing the range of analytical instruments—mainly optical or electronic—used in clinical science. A concluding review draws attention to obstacles of organization and communication now restraining the full utilization of instrument technology in medicine, and identifies some trends and tasks for the future.

CHAPTER 2

THE LIVING MACHINE

In the first chapter the body was described as a power station. The robots of science fiction usually appear to rely on electrical energy, and designers of robot-like machines turn first to familiar electrical power supplies operating conventional electromechanical transducers. The designer of a powered prosthesis to replace a human limb or organ soon realizes that the abilities of such technology compare very unfavourably with what is provided in living organisms. His metallic conductors and solid-state devices are poor substitutes for natural components in the information and control systems of the body. There liquid-state devices are the rule, with membranes in vital roles. Ions moving in electrolytes replace the conduction electrons in metals, and subtle transducers are fed with chemical rather than electrical energy.

The body is thus not amenable to study or testing by techniques which would suffice for an electrical machine. However, certain stages in the functioning of the control mechanisms generate potential differences and provide sufficient electrical energy to give useful data when observed with relatively simple apparatus. In a few instances the natural system may be linked to an electronic device which can supplement or take over a vital function.

In this chapter we outline some of the techniques for studying those bioelectric potentials which give useful information to the clinician, mention some in which the challenge to technology has caused more interest than the results at present justify and discuss one example of therapeutic benefit obtained by linking an electronic instrument to the natural system.

Across the wall of a living cell there is movement of ions due to diffusion and to active transport mechanisms. There is dynamic equilibrium in a resting cell; the concentration of potassium is higher on the inside and the concentration of sodium and chlorine is higher on the outside. This polarization causes a potential difference across the wall or membrane, some 90 mV in a typical muscle cell.

When a nerve or muscle is excited there is a sudden change in the permeability of the membrane. Depolarization occurs, and the potential difference rapidly drops to zero, overshoots and returns to normal more slowly as the membrane repolarizes. In the long fibres, the excitation and the depolarization signal travels along at a speed in

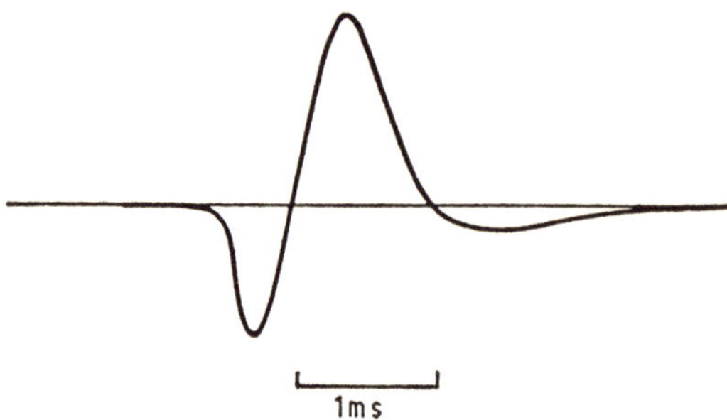

Fig. 1 Action potential of a nerve fibre.

the range of from 1 to 100 m/s. It can be regarded as a moving electric dipole, producing potential changes in the surrounding conducting media. The change (relative to a distant electrode) measured by a small electrode near to the fibre is known as the *action potential*. The typical waveform is illustrated in fig. 1. Action potentials produced by travelling excitations are the source of the potential changes measured in the techniques described in the following paragraphs.

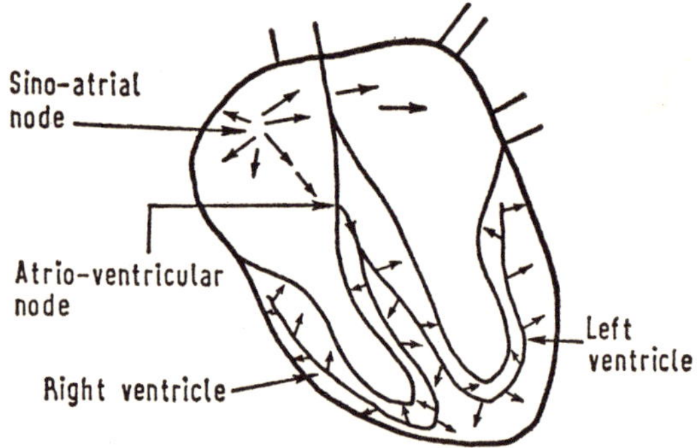

Fig. 2 Spread of excitation through the heart.

Electrocardiography

In the muscles of the heart large numbers of fibres are stimulated and contract almost simultaneously. The resulting potential changes are large enough to be measured at distant points on the surface of the trunk. The trunk acts as a volume conductor; the limbs may be regarded as linear conductors connected to the trunk.

The sino-atrial node (a node is a junction point in a system of fibres) is a region of the atrial wall* which spontaneously depolarizes in a regular manner. It acts as a free-running oscillator, although its

* The atrial wall is the wall of the atrium, the chamber of the heart which empties into the ventricle.

frequency is modified in response to the needs of the body. Excitation here spreads rapidly through the atrium. This will produce a transient potential difference of a few tenths of a millivolt between electrodes on the right arm and left leg. The transient is known as the P wave (fig. 3). The excitation also stimulates the atrio-ventricular node, which delays the passing down of the excitation through a bundle of fibres which branch out and spread it over the large ventricular muscles. This almost simultaneous excitation of many fibres produces the QRS complex (fig. 3). During occurrence of this complex the atria repolarize. A period free from electrical activity is followed by slow repolarization of the ventricles, producing a broad, less defined, T wave (fig. 3). Electrodes in other positions will record the various

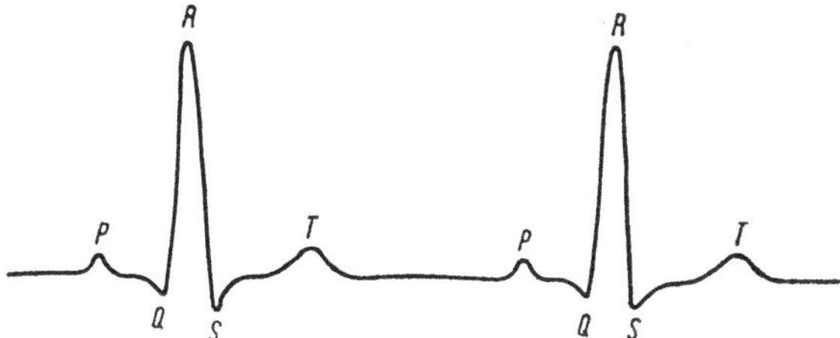

Fig. 3 Normal electrocardiogram for case in which electrodes are sited on right arm and left leg, showing form of P, QRS and T complexes.

phases with different amplitudes. Those close to the heart or inside its chambers will show greater potentials, dominated by the effects of nearer muscles.

This is only a broad outline of the events: to gather detailed information it is usual in *scalar* cardiography* to record potentials using many electrode positions.

The term *lead* is used in a special sense in cardiology:† it refers to the precise arrangement of connexions to the patient which results in the recorded trace. A simple lead is exemplified by one electrode on an arm and the other on a leg. In a complex lead each input terminal of the recorder may be connected to an array of electrodes through resistors. The influence of the lead or connecting system on the waveform recorded may be given a precise mathematical expression, described later in this article.

Twelve standard leads are commonly used. The right leg is used for earthing. The left leg and two arms give three leads. Each of these may also be measured relative to a point which is connected to them through three identical resistors giving *unipolar* leads; others measure potentials on the chest wall relative to the central terminal described,

* Cardiography is the recording of heart variables.
† Cardiology is the knowledge and study of the heart.

or to a terminal connected to two limbs, with or without series resistors.

Experience allows the waveform to be related to anatomical and pathological variations,* but the leads are devised to aid one in rational interpretation of measurements made from the waveforms. For electrodes at these distances the complex electrical dipole pattern can be represented by a single dipole which changes during the cycle. Its axis and dipole moment can be represented by a vector. The effect of the lead, i.e. the electrode positions, on the recorded potential can also be represented by a vector, the *lead vector*. The potential difference recorded at any instant is given by the scalar product of these vectors. For the limb-to-limb leads the situation is illustrated by the simple geometrical construction shown in fig. 4. The lead vectors

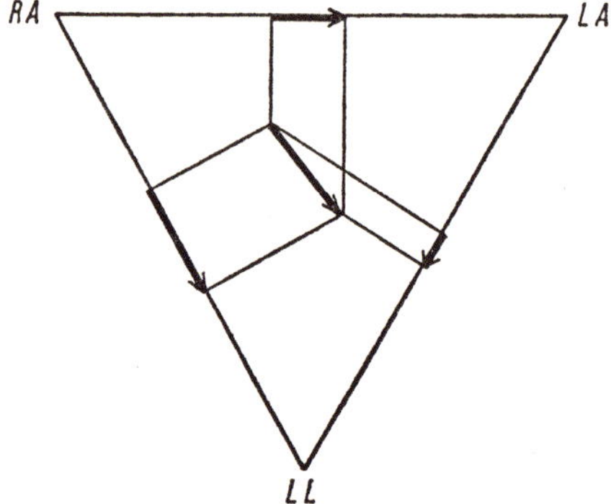

Fig. 4 The Einthoven triangle construction for limb leads.

form an equilateral triangle round the heart and the projection of the heart vector on each shows the relative potentials in these leads. Simultaneous recording of the different leads is desirable, otherwise the information content is degraded.

Electrocardiograms were recorded successfully sixty years ago using string galvanometers. These remarkable instruments were lacking in robustness and convenience and were superseded by mirror galvanometers driven by valve amplifiers: with these instruments there was still delay in processing the light-sensitive paper. When the electrocardiograph (e.c.g.) is used to monitor the general state of the heart and no record is required, e.g. during surgical operations, cathode-ray tube display is excellent. Direct writing is more suitable for the cardiologist; pen or hot-stylus recording is customary. The first recorders used had a poor frequency response: this remains a

* Pathology is the science of disease. Pathological variations are variations due to disease.

limiting factor in some units. Ink-jet writing systems are not limited in the same way. Ultra-violet recorders have not been used to any great extent yet in clinical instruments.

Transistor amplifiers replaced valves when high input impedance became possible. The high impedance is necessary to minimize the adverse effects of the impedance present at the skin connexion. This can decrease signal amplitude and increase the interference picked up by the body-lead loop. It can also introduce serious distortion of the record when the lead system involves a reference point formed by a direct connexion between two limbs, for then inequalities of imped-ance at the limbs may change the lead vector and thus affect the amplitude of some waves: serious errors in diagnosis may result. The deliberate addition of series resistors sufficient to swamp the varia-tions in skin impedance is practicable only if the input impedance is high. Modern instruments have impedances from 1 to 10 MΩ, much superior to those formerly used, but a further order of magnitude is probably desirable and practicable. The usual low frequency res-ponse limit, 0·08 Hz, is satisfactory, but the desirable upper limit is not generally agreed. For some purposes a 3 dB point at 50 Hz may be sufficient, but when a cardiologist wishes to see fine detail in the faster parts of the trace he may require a response substantially flat to several hundred hertz. The discriminating user will ask for a res-ponse curve rather than a statement about a 3 dB or other single point. He will also investigate the linearity of voltage sensitivity across the chart, which is not always satisfactory.

Hospital wards and operating theatres may be very noisy electri-cally (as well as acoustically). Interference picked up in the body, mostly at mains frequency, presents problems. Differential amplifiers are invariably used; a high common mode rejection ratio, say 5000:1, is desirable.

All instruments have calibration facilities, lead selectors and a chart speed of 25 mm/s. Depending on the use and the price range, additional features may include several other speeds, simultaneous recording of several leads and a coding on the record to indicate leads and speeds used. In miniature portable units some technical com-promises may be necessary, e.g. between battery life and the frequency response of the recorder.

Vector cardiography. This approach, more sophisticated than scalar cardiography, produces an analogue display of the movement of the heart vector. Its tip can be imagined to trace a pattern in space which can be projected on to orthogonal planes. The record shows several closed loops, as in fig. 5. The ideal planes are vertical (frontal), sagittal* and transverse. If leads with vectors directed orthogonally in these planes were used and the signals applied to the X and Y

* A sagittae plane is anterior-posterior, parallel to the long axis of the body.

plates of a cathode-ray tube, the loops in the plane defined by the two leads would be shown. Trace modulation can be used for time indication. The chief difficulty of vector cardiology lies in producing leads with these vectors for all positions and conditions of the heart.

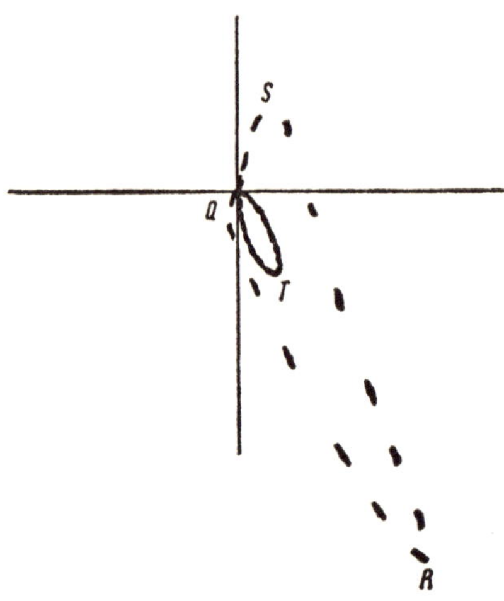

Fig. 5 Vector cardiogram of *QRS* and *T* complexes (see fig. 3), frontal plane.

Leads can be studied by supposing that a voltage is applied across the electrodes and considering the electric field through the heart. The ideal lead would give lines of induction parallel to the required plane at all points. Arrays of electrodes have been devised to do this. Amplifiers of the type already described are used with standard techniques for X–Y display.

The vector cardiogram displays all the available electrical information in a vivid form, but the concepts involved are difficult for the cardiologist with little scientific training. As a routine diagnostic aid it has not been widely used.

Vector cardiology has now been overtaken by the possibilities of computer analysis of data. Simultaneous recordings of orthogonal leads have been shown to contain the information in the most economical manner, and to be the most reliable for diagnosis. The computer can deal with the cardiologist's main problem, which lies not in the collection of the data but in the evaluation of the large amount of information given by a few seconds of recording. By computer studies the diagnostic value of many parameters has been studied: some combinations of vectors derived from orthogonal leads, which could not be derived without the computer, appear to have diagnostic value superior to the parameters used in scalar cardiography. The electrocardiograph of the future may well carry out digital conversion and link directly to a computer. An intermediate stage will probably involve the recording of digital data on magnetic tape.

Foetal electrocardiography

Electrodes placed on the foetal head allow small but complete complexes to be recorded, but this is practicable only at the terminal stage of pregnancy. Electrodes on the maternal abdomen show signals at a remarkably early stage (sometimes at the end of the third month, almost always by the fifth month). The signal is small—the R wave (see fig. 3) may be from 5 to 25 μV—and is superimposed on a larger maternal electrocardiogram and mixed with irregular signals from muscle which at best are a little smaller than the R wave and at worst

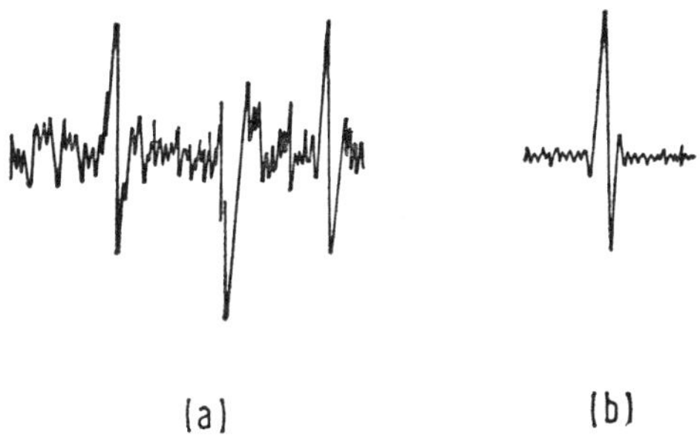

(a)   (b)

Fig. 6 Foetal electrocardiogram: (*left*) single trace and (*right*) average of many traces.

are much larger. The muscle noise is the most troublesome: a computer of average transients, or other device for extracting signal from noise, is essential if more than the peak of the R wave is to be seen (fig. 6). The information gleaned from R wave alone is not sufficient to justify the difficult exercise.

A discouraging feature of foetal electrocardiography is that it unpredictably fails to produce any result at times, even in a normal subject studied successfully at other times. The extraction of the full electrocardiogram is a challenge, but its value in clinical practice cannot yet be predicted.

Electro-encephalography

A multitude of nerve cells in the brain produces action potentials. There is no simple synchronization comparable with that of the heart, but electrodes placed on the scalp or inserted into the surface of the cortex (the convoluted outer layer of the brain) record potentials with low-frequency variations. The voltage, peak to peak, is usually below 100 μV and waveforms are roughly sinusoidal. The frequency and amplitude vary with the general level of cerebral activity. Detail varies over the cortex: since the influence of the nearest areas predominates, pathological changes which affect the electrical activity can be localized. An array of many leads is generally used and signals from eight to sixteen electrodes simultaneously recorded relative to a distant electrode. Studies are made of activity both spontaneous and stimulated (e.g. by flashing light).

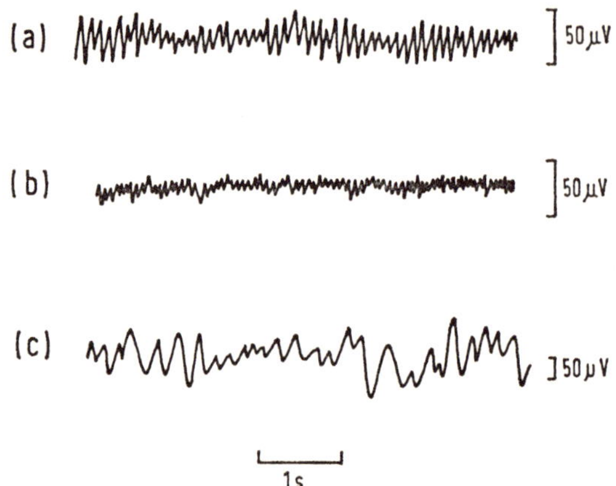

Fig. 7 Electro-encephalograms: (*a*) alpha rhythm, (*b*) beta rhythm and (*c*) delta rhythm.

Certain significant though not completely distinct parts of the frequency spectrum are recognized. The so-called alpha rhythms, with frequencies of 8 to 13 Hz, predominate in a relaxed state. Excitement produces the more rapid beta and gamma rhythms, deep sleep or anaesthesia the slow delta and theta rhythms (see fig. 7). Characteristic changes occur in the epileptic subject, and several other abnormal conditions can be diagnosed. In research on the brain the recording of these rhythms—electro-encephalography—is invaluable.

The wide range of signals, from 5 μV upwards, fed to an electro-encephalograph (e.e.g.) necessitates an amplifier with a sensitivity of 10 μV/cm and a good attenuation range. Low noise level is essential: it is normally less than 2 μV peak to peak with 5 kΩ input load. As in the e.c.g., high input impedance is required: values of over 10 MΩ are obtainable. A common mode rejection ratio of at least 1000:1 at mains frequency is required: some instruments offer ten times as much. There are usually ranges of time constant and high-frequency cut-off filters. Paper speeds should include 1·5, 3 and 6 cm/s.

Upwards of twenty electrodes may be attached to the patient and a master pattern selector is advantageous. The resistance at each electrode must be monitored for otherwise an artefact due to high resistance might be interpreted as significant. It is normal to provide a meter, but one make of machine permits the measurement of eight resistances simultaneously, the results being recorded on the paper. The same model also indicates on the record the electrode pattern, voltage sensitivity, time constant and high-frequency cut-off. One manufacturer provides for the measurement of the rejection ratio of each channel. Ink recorders are usually used: linearity is less important than for the e.c.g. as precise potential measurement is not meaningful.

Most instruments are now fully transistorized, although some are still made with valve pre-amplifiers. The consequent improvement of reliability is welcome, for experience with the previous generation of valve instruments was often unhappy. However, faults were not always due to valves or other components of expectedly short life; they were sometimes in selector switches or other parts, not easily or quickly replaceable. Purchasers may be greatly influenced by the thought given to speedy fault elimination, availability of replacement modules and by servicing arrangements in general.

Information from the electro-encephalogram is even more difficult to interpret than from the electrocardiogram. Significant patterns may appear at irregular intervals on long records and may involve changes in several channels which cannot be detected by eye. Digital computers are applied, but until they have contributed more to basic research on the origins of e.c.g. signals the extent of their routine clinical use is not likely to be significant.

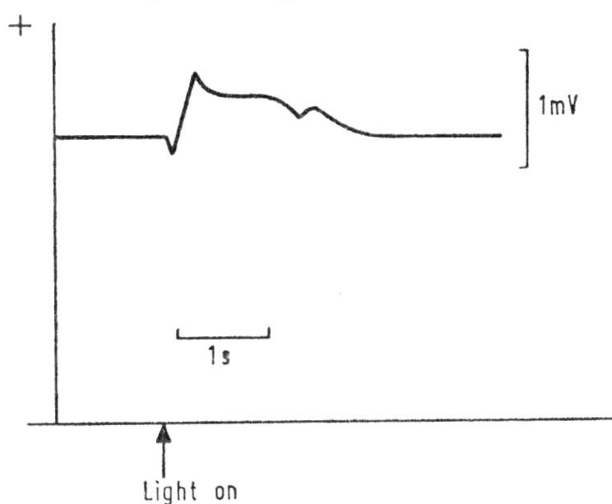

Fig. 8 Electroretinogram.

Electroretinography and electro-oculography

All sense organs are connected to the brain but the eye has a special relationship as the retina is an extension of the cerebral cortex. Potentials within the eye may be recorded relatively easily because of its exposed position.

The cornea is about 20 mV positive relative to the fundus* of the eye. If the illumination of the retina is changed the potential changes slightly in a complex manner. The recording of these changes is called the electroretinogram (fig. 8). A silver chloride electrode on a contact lens and a 'distant' electrode on the cheek are used. The largest variations are usually slightly less than 1 mV. The technique is not used very much clinically but is of value in research on vision and some disorders which affect it: electroencephalographic or similar equipment is usually available and serves adequately for recording.

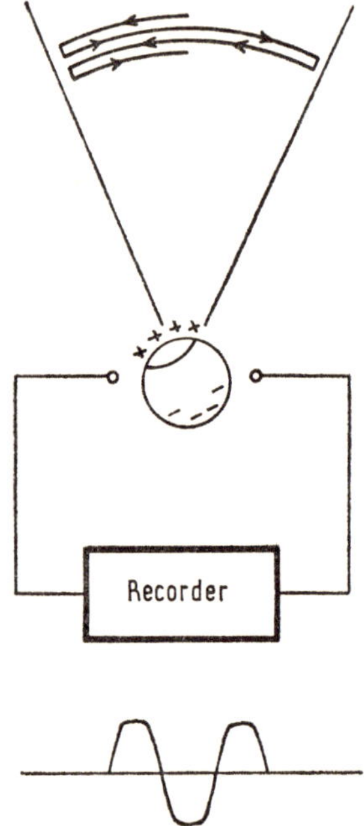

Fig. 9 How an electro-oculogram is recorded.

The steady potential may be studied by the simple technique of electro-oculography. Skin electrodes are placed on either side of the eye, which is then rhythmically rotated as the vision shifts between two fixation points (fig. 9). An alternating potential difference of 1 mV or more is recorded. Some diseases which affect the steady potential may be usefully studied. Similar principles are applied when the movements of the eye are under investigation.

Electromyography

Diseases which affect the skeletal muscles can be investigated by observing the action potentials of muscle fibres. Limited data are

* The fundus is the back of the interior of the eyeball.

available from surface electrodes; more use is made of needle electrodes inserted into the muscle. The measurements made may be of
potentials between the needle tip and a surface electrode, or between
two or more electrodes introduced at the tip of a thin cannula.*
Depending on the size and position of the electrodes, action potentials from a few or many motor units may be observed. The motor
units comprise muscle fibres simultaneously excited by a nerve. Contractions of different motor units are not synchronized. The overall
number excited per second increases with increasing effort of the
muscle.

The waveforms normally recorded are similar to the action potential form of fig. 1. The repetition frequency may vary widely from a
few per second in resting muscle to hundreds per second when many
motor units are firing. The rise time of the spike is a small fraction of a
millisecond, and the limits of amplifier frequency response (3 dB
points) should not be narrower than 2 to 10000 Hz if full value is to
be obtained from the record. In general this implies cathode-ray tube
presentation, although for some purposes the limits imposed by pen
recording may be acceptable. The c.r.t. is used for observation and is
photographed for records.

A better but more expensive method of recording is on magnetic
tape, preferably with a frequency modulation system. The signal is
also fed to a loudspeaker, and the characteristic sound is as useful to
the experienced operator as the visual display. Since the impedances
of the small electrodes may be very high, approaching a megohm, a
high-impedance input is again essential. The input lead to ground
capacitance must also be small. Relatively large potentials are produced by needle movements, and overloading and blocking of the
amplifier may result: a compromise between low frequency response
and blocking time is necessary. A useful sensitivity range is 50 μV/cm
to 5 mV/cm, with sweep speeds in the region of 1 mm/ms.

Multichannel instruments are available: some have separate tubes
for viewing and recording, with variable film speed, automatic trace
brightness control and similar features. As well as recording during
natural contraction one studies the response to electrical stimulation,
and facilities are provided for synchronizing the sweep with the
applied stimulus.

Heart stimulation

The contraction produced by electrical stimulation of muscle gives
rise to several medical instruments. Brief reference is made here to
only one application, namely the production of useful contractions
in the heart ventricles. This may be needed when the heart action has
ceased, e.g. following coronary thrombosis, or when the excitation is

* A cannula is a small tube normally used for draining fluids.

not being conducted from the pacemaker to the ventricular muscles.

Another condition amenable to electrical correction is ventricular fibrillation—a state in which the muscle fibres contract not synchronously, but irregularly, with results which may be fatal. Fibrillation may be cured by giving the muscle an electric shock. This is not too difficult if the heart is exposed, say when the fibrillation occurs during an operation (internal defibrillation). It is more difficult to deliver the shock through the intact chest wall (external defibrillation). Some defibrillators apply an alternating voltage. Between 1 and 5 A should pass through the heart, which offers an impedance of 20 to 50 Ω. Some internal defibrillators use a series resistance to swamp the variable heart impedance, others allow adjustment dependent on preliminary resistance measurement with a small applied voltage. If electrodes are applied externally, perhaps a fifth of the current passes through the heart and the impedance may be almost 100Ω. The very high voltages necessary in these circumstances can cause severe burns at the skin surface if contact resistance is high. In practice the voltage is usually restricted to less than a thousand and in some cases the resulting currents may be too small.

No further development of a.c. instruments seems profitable, for it is believed that direct current produced by condenser discharge is more effective, i.e. less energy is required. Both energy and current waveform seem to be important, though the relevant parameters are not satisfactorily established. Quoted values of optimum energy differ by factors of five, the maxima being about 75 joules for internal application and 250 for external. The addition of inductance to give a slightly oscillatory discharge seems to improve the efficiency. Condensers used have generally been of 16 μF; the weight is appreciable. In order to use electrolytic capacitors one circuit employs low voltage and high capacitance, discharging through an impulse transformer to obtain the equivalent of a high-voltage low-capacitance output. There are other types of fibrillation or irregular rhythm where the shocks should be synchronized with any spontaneous electrocardiographic signals: this facility is now provided in most d.c. defibrillators.

When all heart activity ceases, or when the normal pacing signal fails to reach the ventricles, artificial pacemaking is required. In the first minutes of the emergency a voltage applied through external electrodes may supply sufficient energy to trigger the ventricles. The source should supply from 15 to 100 V at 200 mA maximum, in rounded pulses lasting 2 or 3 ms, at a repetition frequency around 60/min.

For periods of a few days the heart can be paced using an external pulse generator and electrodes inserted into the heart through veins. Pulses of 2 ms are satisfactory; the voltage required is usually less than 5 but some margin should be provided. Problems of infection limit the duration of use of such a method and for long-term pacing the entire apparatus should be implanted.

Much publicity has been accorded to implanted pacemakers: they have caught the layman's imagination. It is perhaps justifiable to strike a cautious (or even slightly sour) note in correction of the tendency for self-congratulation on the part of users or makers of these devices. When satisfactory they are life-giving aids almost magical in apparent simplicity, but the failure rate is deplorable at the present time. It is to be expected that the battery may be a weak item in the pulse generator, but failures due to other component or connexion faults in the encapsulated pulse generator are not rare. A user who does careful tests can spot some of these before insertion. Fluids still leak in after implantation, and fracture of leads due to the regular movement of the heart remains a problem despite many and considerable improvements in their design. A team which brought the best modern engineering to bear on pacemaker design might not share the applause accorded—rightly—to the pioneers, but it would save many lives.

CHAPTER 3

GATHERING DATA WITH THE HELP OF TRANSDUCERS

A transducer as it is understood in medicine is a device which receives a signal in one form of energy and converts that signal into a different form of energy. Transducers provide signals which are related in a known way to parameters which it is desired to measure. Taking temperature as an example, a frequently used transducer is the thermocouple, which provides an electromotive force very nearly proportional to the difference between the measured temperature and a standard temperature, say that of a flask of melting ice. Transducers having, like the thermocouple, an electrical output, are preferred in many applications—especially where amplification or automatic recording of the transducer signal is required. However, despite the increasingly dominant position occupied by electronics in the measurement field, transducers heed not have this kind of output. I shall describe later some interesting examples of transducers which are basically non-electronic in operation.

Patient and transducer

Apart from purely instrumental considerations, the desirable properties of a transducer for making physiological measurements on a patient are influenced by the special nature of the relationship between the patient and the transducer. The application of transducers to the patient may reasonably be tolerated only if certain requirements are met. For the anaesthetized or unconscious patient this is mainly a question of avoiding all unnecessary injury; for the conscious, however, the transducer must also be as unobtrusive and unrestrictive as possible. In the latter case, especially, this may mean that the transducer is operating under difficult conditions involving a poor signal/noise ratio.

The measurement of blood pressure is a good example. When it is possible, as in the operating theatre, to connect a manometer directly to the blood supply, the principal difficulties are those of access and blood clotting. However, when, as in the ward or consulting room, an inflatable arm cuff is used to occlude (obstruct) the blood vessels, determination of blood pressure depends on the ability to recognize at what point in the deflation of the arm cuff the arterial blood flow resumes. The trained ear of a physician listening with a stethoscope placed over the brachial artery (the arm artery) discriminates the significant sounds from a medley of irrelevant noise created by slight patient movements, not to mention external background. If this could be done automatically, then measurement could be very frequent and personal bias would be eliminated, but a simple microphone followed by an electronic amplitude discriminator falls far short of what is required to make automation possible.

The relationship between clinician – be he surgeon or physician – and transducer must also be considered. The clinician is expected to tolerate the presence of transducers, but he is in a position of responsibility and command, and he will rightly object to a transducer which, while causing much inconvenience, provides little, irrelevant or superflous information. For example, if relative values have much more significance than high absolute accuracies, there is no point in complicating matters to achieve the latter. Again, even supposing that the transducer is well designed for the measurement it has to make, its signals may be of little value to the clinician unless correspondingly good design has gone into the instrumentation which processes them.

Measurable parameters

A wide variety of physiological parameters is open to measurement by means of transducers. Pressure, flow and total volume of blood in the circulatory system, and also pulse rate, may each be ascertained by several methods. The same is true for the corresponding quantities associated with the respiratory system. Temperature is an easy parameter to measure, especially by electronic means, and may be monitored in almost any part of the body.

By way of contrast, body kinetics have been studied for the most part by relatively crude methods. With the development of miniature displacement and acceleration transducers, more refined observations will be increasingly possible. Such properties of body fluids as pH, the partial pressure of oxygen and carbon dioxide (P_{O_2} and P_{CO_2}) and viscosity may be measured *in vivo*, although the accuracies possible are often much less than if the fluid were isolated from the body. For measurements in inaccessible parts of the body advantage may sometimes be taken of telemetry and the radio pill. The radio link also has important possibilities for monitoring physiological functions during physical activity.

The circulatory system consists of the heart, with the arteries, veins and capillaries which carry the blood to and from the lungs and to and from the rest of the body. The study of pressure and flow patterns within this system can be of great significance in the diagnosis of abnormal conditions, especially those involving defects of the heart itself or of the large arteries and veins.

Pressure measurements

The most direct method of measuring blood pressure would be to insert into a blood vessel a tube of convenient diameter and connect it to a U-tube manometer. This kind of procedure could, of course, only be used under sterile conditions and would be suitable mainly for the operating theatre. A fluid-filled manometer of this type would certainly be too sluggish to follow accurately the pressure variations occurring during the pumping cycle of the heart. A pressure transducer of the capacitive, inductive or strain gauge type is better. The system is still fluid-filled, for the physiological reason that gas bubbles must be kept out of the blood stream and for the physical reason that frequency response must be adequate. The role of the saline-filled U-tube is relegated to that of providing a check on the overall gain of the system.

The places at which it is convenient to insert a tube, or catheter as it is called, into an artery or vein are not generally those at which pressure measurements are most needed. However, with the help of combined X-ray and television techniques, the position of the catheter tip may be easily followed as it advances along an appropriate artery or vein of an arm or leg. In this way pressure may be monitored at any desired point in the great blood vessels or the chambers of the heart. In general, the right-hand side of the heart (which pumps the blood to the lungs) may be reached through a vein while the left-hand side (which pumps the blood round the rest of the body) may be reached through an artery.

There are two important limitations on the accuracy of measuring pressure by means of the saline-filled catheter and external pressure transducer. The first follows from the fact that the catheter is effectively a lossy transmission line terminated with a large reactance. Best results are obtained when the large reactance, that is to say the transducer, is placed in parallel with a needle-valve leak which may be varied so as to equal the catheter's characteristic resistance. Unfortunately this point may not be widely appreciated, and, moreover, the device leads to practical complications since steps must be taken to prevent blocking of the needle valve by clotting blood. Typically it is possible to record with fidelity up to about 100 Hz, but the frequency limit is much lower with the narrower catheters that sometimes must be used, too low in fact to give pressure waveforms of diagnostic value. The other limitation is that the pumping action of the heart can cause quite considerable movements of the catheter tip and these are recorded as spurious pressure fluctuations.

Improvements are possible by using a miniature pressure transducer mounted on the catheter tip. Such a transducer is the Allard–Laurens micromanometer. It is of the variable-inductance type, its

B

external shape being a cylinder 2·7 mm in diameter and 8 mm long. Still more miniaturization would be needed before this type of transducer could be mounted on even the largest catheters which it is possible to use for small infants, so here again catheter diameter is a serious limitation.

Indirect measurement of pressure

Blood pressure is measured indirectly by means of an inflatable cuff encircling a limb, usually the upper arm. Although the detailed shape of the pressure waveform cannot be followed by this method, it is possible to determine the systolic (maximum) and diastolic (minimum) arterial pressures.

The cuff is first inflated to a pressure above the systolic so that the blood flow is completely occluded. The cuff pressure is then allowed to fall slowly. Once it is below the systolic pressure there is an intermittent flow of blood through the arteries. The flow becomes continuous when the diastolic pressure is passed. During the period of intermittent flow, the rhythmic collapsing of the arterial walls under the pressure of the cuff gives rise to a characteristic noise known as the Korotkoff sounds, which can be heard with the aid of a stethoscope. Unfortunately the pressure exerted on the limb by the cuff is slightly less than the pressure within the cuff, the excess being larger for narrower cuffs (the higher pressure is due to tension in the cuff wall, and is analogous to the excess pressure contained by surface tension in a bubble or droplet). A large cuff of standard size is therefore used whenever possible, so that measurements are strictly comparable whether they are taken with an automatic apparatus or with a simple hand-operated sphygmomanometer.

The inadequacy of the microphone (when compared with the trained ear) for detecting the Korotkoff sounds has already been mentioned. A way of overcoming the difficulty is to gate the microphone so that its output is only accepted during that fraction of the heart cycle in which the Korotkoff sounds occur. The gating signal may, for example, be derived from an auxiliary transducer picking up a pulse signal from a finger of the opposite arm.

A more fundamental solution, which liberates an automatic system from the danger of responding to background sounds, lies in the detection of the phenomena which give rise to the Korotkoff sounds, that is to say, the rhythmic volume changes of the arteries during the period of intermittent blood flow. Fig. 10 shows diagrammatically a sophisticated double-cuff arrangement which does just this. The upper and lower parts of the cuff, labelled A and B respectively, communicate with the two compression chambers, C_1 and C_2. The arterial volume changes cause in A and B corresponding volume changes which in turn cause jets of air to pass into the compression chambers.

The presence of the jets is detected by the thermistors T_1 and T_2 in the following way. As the cuff pressure drops below the systolic and the first volume of blood passes under both parts of the cuff, T_1 receives a puff of air in C_1 and is cooled. From this is derived the command signal to record the systolic pressure. During the interval of intermittent flow between the systolic and diastolic pressures the

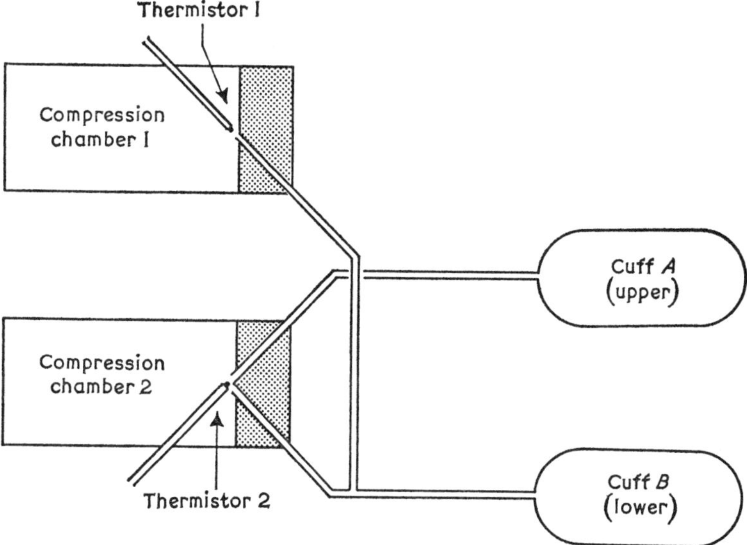

Fig. 10 Simplified diagram of double arm-cuff transducer system of Godart Haemotonograph automatic blood pressure recorder. (*Courtesy of Godart C.P.I. Ltd.*)

arrival in C_2 of a puff of air from A precedes the arrival of the corresponding puff B by an appreciable fraction of a second; the puff from A has time to cool T_2 before being blown off course by the puff from B, and from this a signal is derived. The situation alters as the cuff pressure drops below the diastolic. The blood flow becomes continuous, and the interval between the arrival times of the two air puffs in C_2 becomes less than a millisecond, with the result that T_2 is no longer cooled. The command signal to record diastolic pressure is therefore generated by the cessation of signals from T_2.

Measurement of blood flow

Blood flow turns out to be much more difficult to measure than blood pressure. Even for blood flow in an external circuit, like that of a heart-lung machine, flowmeters with sharp edges or moving parts are unacceptable because of the damage they cause to the blood cells. In an intact vessel the situation is further complicated by the inclusion within the flow transducer of the vessel walls; this introduces a number of unknown and varying quantities quite apart from the blood flow to be measured.

Because of certain theoretical advantages, such as linearity of response to both magnitude and direction of flow and negligible disturbance to the measured flow, the electromagnetic type of flowmeter has been much studied. The transducer has to be matched to the blood vessel so that the latter fits snugly in the opening for it.

Essentially the transducer is an electromagnet with a pair of electrodes to pick up potentials induced by the flow of an electrically conducting fluid within the magnetic field.

The flow-induced signal is exactly proportional to the magnetic field, and, for all practical purposes, proportional to the volume rate of flow through the transducer. The reason for having an electromagnet rather than a permanent magnet is that an a.c. system is required for the elimination of thermo-electric and electrochemical potentials. The current exciting the electromagnet may be either square or sinusoidal in waveform, unique advantages being claimed for each. The main point about square-wave excitation is that the pick-up electrode may be gated so that only the flow-induced potentials are measured, while potentials induced by variation of the magnetic field ('transformer effect') are automatically excluded.

Pulse rate measurement

Pulse rate may be derived from the pressure or flow waveforms, or an electrocardiograph can be used. However, one of the neatest ways of detecting the pulse is by the use of a miniature light source and photocell to detect the variation of transmitted light through the finger pulp as the blood flushes through the capillaries.

Ratemeters of the diode pump type are not well suited to the measurement of rates like that of the pulse, which are of the order of one event per second. An alternative is to measure the time interval between successive pulse signals and to follow this with a time-to-rate converter (i.e. a simple analogue computer which finds the reciprocal). Generally accuracy better than about 2 per cent is not needed and quite simple circuitry is adequate.

Blood volume and cardiac output

The cardiac output is the volume of blood which the heart pumps in unit time to either the body or the lungs. For a normal human heart the two volume rates of flow are equal. Where there is a 'hole in the heart' some of the oxygenated blood being pumped to the body can be mixed with carbon dioxide-laden blood going to the lungs. In this case the concept of cardiac output is not so simply defined.

If a quantity of an indicating substance—for example, a harmless dye—is injected into a vein a short distance from the heart, its distribution through an artery may be followed in space and time. It is then possible to estimate both the total blood volume and the cardiac output. Fig. 11 shows an indicator dilution curve on a normal subject. The detector in this case is a photo-electric transducer, clipped to the ear lobe, which senses increased absorption in the red and infra-red parts of the spectrum on passage of the dye. There is a time lag

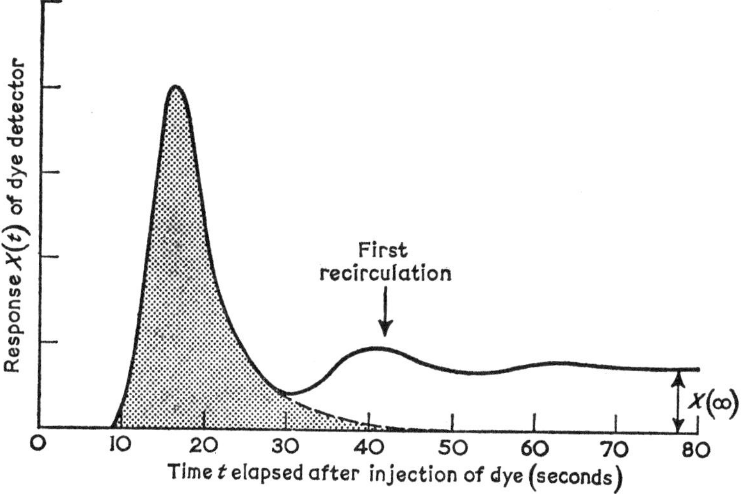

Fig. 11 Typical indicator dilution curve on a normal subject. Indicating dye is injected at $t = 0$ into a large vein.

('appearance time') between injection and the first detection of the indicator because the first circulation flow is through the lungs. The curve clearly shows how quickly the indicator is mixed throughout the whole blood volume; in fact, the peak corresponding to the first recirculation is well down compared with the maximum detected concentration, while the peak corresponding to the second recirculation is hardly discernible.

If the detector has been designed so that its response X is proportional to the concentration C of the indicator in the blood, then the total blood volume V is given by—

$$I = VC_\infty = VX_\infty/\alpha$$

where I is the total amount of the indicator, C_∞ and X_∞ are respectively the indicator concentration and the detector response after complete mixing, and α is a calibration factor determined by withdrawing a blood sample so that C_∞ may be measured directly.

In the absence of recirculation the cardiac output F would be related to I by the equation—

$$I = \frac{F}{\alpha} \int_0^\infty X_t \, dt$$

where X_t is the indicator response at time t. In the practical case the first fall of the curve is assumed to be exponential and is extrapolated as shown by the dashed line in fig. 11. The integral is then represented by the shaded area. Cardiac output computers, now available commercially, automatically integrate the appropriate part of the indicator

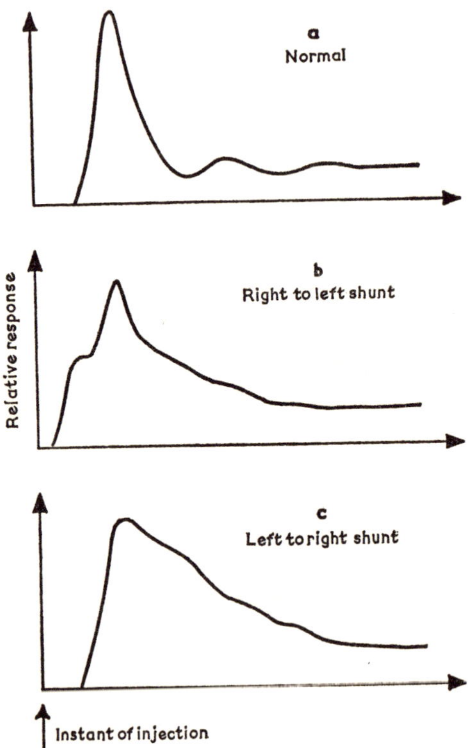

Fig. 12 Effect of 'hole in the heart' on indicator dilution curve.

dilution curve signal and give a direct reading of cardiac output. Fig. 12 shows two typical ways in which a 'hole in the heart' may affect the indicator dilution curve. Although in these cases cardiac output is not meaningfully defined by the above equation, the shape of the curve, especially the position of the peaks, is of diagnostic value.

The interesting physiological parameters of the respiratory system are basically the same as those of the circulatory system, namely pressure, flows and volumes. There is obviously a difference in dealing with a gas rather than a liquid. Also the lungs (unlike the heart) are partially under voluntary control. Thus there is dissimilarity between the transducer systems required for respiratory and circulatory measurements. Indeed, owing to the desirability of simultaneously determining physical and biochemical parameters, the modern tendency is towards apparatus which records not only the volumes and

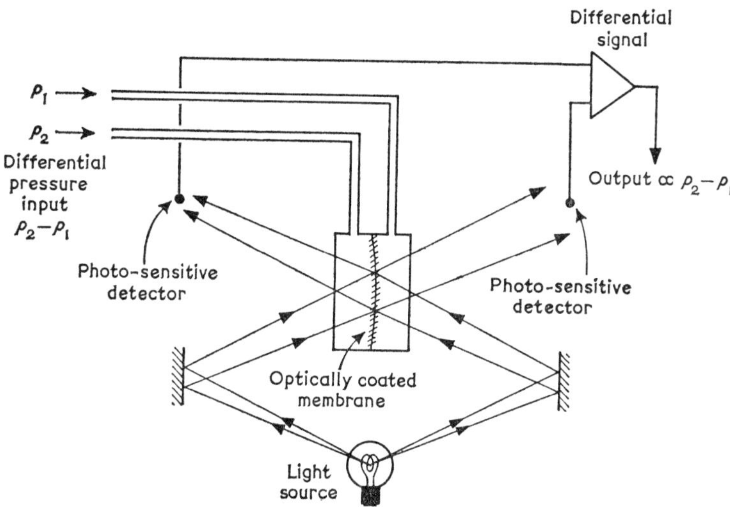

Fig. 13 Diagram showing principle of Greer micromanometer.

pressures involved in respiration but also does continuous chemical analysis of the expired air. However, in this chapter attention will be confined to the transducer systems associated with the physical aspects of lung function.

In general the pressure transducers need to be more sensitive than the capacitive, inductive or strain-gauge types already mentioned. A transducer possessing the sensitivity required in this lower pressure range is the optical focusing/defocusing type used in the Greer micromanometer. The principle is shown diagrammatically in fig. 13. The pressure-sensing diaphragm is optically coated and behaves as a mirror of variable focal length mounted at the centre of a symmetrical optical system. Two phototransistors monitor the focusing effect of the mirror on two beams of light and provide a differential signal which is proportional to the pressure difference. Provided that it is possible to keep the system completely gas-filled, such an arrangement typically has an upper frequency cut-off whose

3 dB point is 100 Hz. Unfortunately the high-frequency response may be sacrificed if parts of the system have to be liquid-filled; in such instances a more conventional transducer with a completely liquid-filled system may be preferable.

Pressures may be of direct interest, for example, where it is desired to measure the resistance to airflow of the airways leading to the lungs. However, the particular value of the Greer micromanometer is realized where very small pressure differences are obtained from a

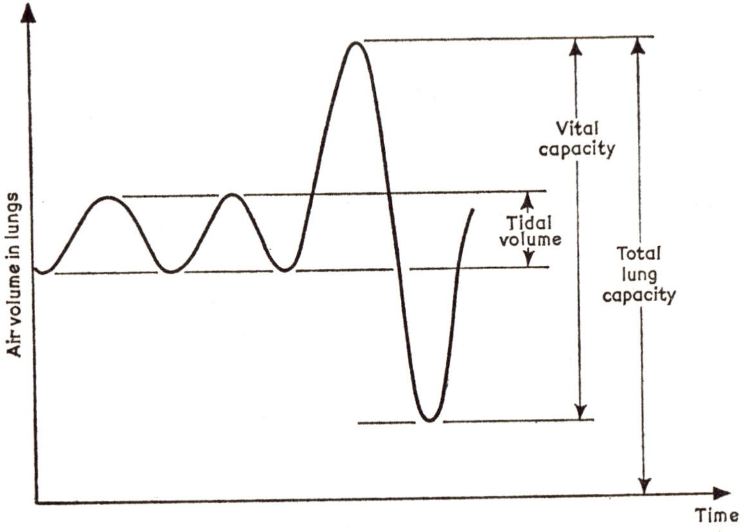

Fig. 14 Variation of lung volume during normal and deep breathing.

transducer which measures flow rate or volume change. Obvious examples are the Pitot tube and the Venturi tube, although they are not useful for measuring airflow into and out of the lungs since they are not suitable for both positive and negative flows. The basis of a suitable transducer is a resistive obstruction, of wire gauze or similar material, which causes a pressure change whose sign corresponds to the flow direction. With correct design the obstruction does not significantly impede the airflow, and the differential pressure output, though small, is proportional to the rate of flow. It is evident that electronic integration of this rate-of-flow signal can provide data on lung volume changes.

Fig. 14 shows lung volume (plotted as a function of time) during normal breathing, followed by a deep breath in and out. Of special clinical interest is the ratio of the volume change in normal breathing ('tidal volume') to the maximum volume change possible with deep breathing in and out ('vital capacity'). The maximum possible lung volume ('total lung capacity') is also of interest, but its measurement requires direct measurement of lung volume (rather than of change in lung volume).

A transducer capable of measuring lung volume as well as change in lung volume is the whole-body plethysmograph. This is a large airtight box which totally encloses the subject, who breathes through a wide-bore tube which passes out of the box. Changes in lung volume are then related by Boyle's law to the associated small pressure changes within the box. Further application of Boyle's law to the case where the wide-bore tube is closed and the subject alters the pressure in it by the effort of his lungs, allows the total lung volume to be found from the changes in the box pressure and the closed tube pressure. Still more information can be found; as a result of the airway resistance, the rate of flow of air to and from the lungs lags slightly behind the changes in lung volume; a dynamic analysis of the relation between rate of flow and lung volume therefore enables one to calculate airway resistance.

A disadvantage of the body plethysmograph for finding total lung volume is that the volume so determined includes all gas trapped in the thorax in addition to the ventilated volume of the lungs. The latter can be found by an indicator dilution technique using an inert gas, such as helium, as indicator in a closed rebreathing apparatus of known volume.

Temperature measurement

The search here is not for a replacement for the mercury-in-glass clinical thermometer, which for use in the ward is convenient, accurate and cheap. The need for continuous temperature monitoring occurs (*a*) in the intensive care of seriously ill patients and (*b*) during and after major surgery in which the patient has been deliberately cooled in order to slow down the life processes.

For such continuous monitoring, transducers having an electrical output are the most suitable and have gained wide acceptance. The resistance thermometer is the most accurate of them; indeed, the platinum resistance thermometer is one of the secondary temperature standards. Nevertheless, the resistance thermometer does not lend itself to incorporation into a small probe, and its inherent absolute accuracy is unnecessary in the clinical field.

In contrast with the resistance thermometer, both the thermocouple and the thermistor are possible transducers for very small probes. It is feasible, for example, to incorporate them in the tip of a narrow hypodermic needle.

Thermocouples are perhaps the more accurate, but, owing to their low output (and the consequent need for d.c. amplification of signal), the tendency is not to use them unless several channels are being monitored in sequence. The disadvantage of a thermostatically controlled oven or ice flask for the reference junction is usually overcome by using instead some form of temperature-sensitive bridge circuit.

Thermistors are resistance elements with a high negative temperature coefficient of resistance and as such require at most a simple Wheatstone bridge circuit and a galvanometric recorder. Moreover, thermistors can now be produced with characteristics closely enough specified to avoid calibration complications. For a single temperature channel a thermistor probe is a cheap and usually completely adequate solution.

The thermistor is a suitable temperature sensor for a telemetering capsule or 'radio pill'. An alternative is to use the marked temperature dependence of germanium transistor characteristics to combine the functions of transducer and oscillator-transmitter. Using a 'radio pill' it is a simple matter to follow the temperature through the entire gastro-intestinal tract.

One of the more elegant ways of studying the body in action is by means of cinematography, usually in slow motion, so that the eye can more readily take in details. Some crude methods have also been used: for example, tremor activity has been measured by the speed with which sand leaves a fenestrated cup subjected to the tremor. Between these extremes of elegance and crudity could lie displacement and acceleration transducers sufficiently small and light not to upset the very aspects of body kinetics they set out to measure, but there has been up to now a dearth of such sensors. A further difficulty is that many of the smaller transducers available (of the piezo-electric type, for instance) are not particularly well suited to the low frequencies met with in physiological recording.

A small acceleration transducer was recently made available by the Ether company with physiological applications in mind. It employs a two-arm semi-conductor strain-gauge bridge actuated by a clamped cantilevered mass, its total weight being only $2\frac{1}{4}$ grammes.

An alternative is a capacitive transducer, which is neater to use in telemetering circuits since it makes possible a frequency-modulated transmitter consisting of a simple transistor oscillator with the transducer as its active element. Such a telemetering device has been used to monitor hand tremor and so assess the value of drug therapy in Parkinson's disease, a disorder of the central nervous system. The transducer was home-made, consisting essentially of a metal plate supported by a phosphor-bronze torsion strip inside a specially shaped box—not unlike the arrangement in the old-fashioned quadrant electrometer, but more robust.

Measurement of the speed and nature of muscle reflexes can be of significance in diagnosing certain metabolic abnormalities. An example is an angular-displacement transducer which is used to measure the 'angle jerk' which occurs when the Achilles tendon is tapped. This is helpful in diagnosing certain disorders of the thyroid gland.

The words 'blood chemistry' conjure up a vision of an extensive field of qualitative investigation and quantitative measurement. While this is not untrue, there are three quantities which it is specially important to be able to measure. These are the partial pressures of oxygen and carbon dioxide in the blood, generally denoted by P_{O_2} and P_{CO_2} and measured in millimetres of mercury, and the acidity or alkalinity of the blood, expressed as hydrogen ion concentration (pH).

Direct determination of P_{O_2}, P_{CO_2} and pH require fairly sophisticated techniques of physical chemistry. The easiest to measure is pH, but since an aqueous carbon dioxide solution is weakly acidic, the pH of blood depends among other things on P_{CO_2}. This means that one really needs simultaneous knowledge of both.

Purpose-made instruments are now available which, from a small blood sample, can quickly provide an anaesthetist with values of P_{O_2}, P_{CO_2} and pH. Oxygen partial pressure is measured by means of a polarographic platinum electrode and a reference electrode in an electrolyte solution, separated from the sample by a permeable polythene membrane. The pH is measured with a sensitive glass electrode in the sample itself, while two further pH determinations, obtained when the sample is divided and mixed with two different known amounts of carbon dioxide, enable one to find P_{CO_2} graphically.

An alternative approach to the oxygen content of the blood is colorimetry, used in this instance to determine the fraction of the haemoglobin combined with oxygen. The brighter red colour of oxyhaemoglobin compared with haemoglobin is due to its weaker absorption in the spectral region from 600 to 800 mμm. If the absorption of transmitted light through a blood sample is measured at two different wavelengths within this spectral range, and the absorption coefficients of haemoglobin and oxyhaemoglobin are known at these two wavelengths, the concentrations of the two substances may be calculated.

The principle of the practical technique is simpler than this because it has been found that, if reflected rather than transmitted light is measured, the absorption is substantially independent of the total haemoglobin concentration; that is, the absorption at a given wavelength is a function of just one variable—the ratio of the two concentrations. For the measurement a red filter, with a transmission band approximately between 600 and 700 mμm, is used. Although the method requires calibration it is fast and reliable. A further advantage may soon be provided by the extreme smallness of the probe made possible by fibre optic technology.

In a heart investigation it is possible, by withdrawing blood via the catheter into a photometric cell, simultaneously to measure the pressure and oxygen saturation of the blood at any point in the heart. The special significance of the catheter is its ability to locate places where the oxygenated blood from the lungs is mixing abnormally with the reduced blood from the rest of the body.

After surveying the wealth of information a clinician can obtain about his patient with the help of transducers it is appropriate to ask to what extent the actual range of the information is limited by the unavailability of suitable transducers. Large size, or an involved procedure for taking readings, may not only make a transducer inconvenient but may completely exclude its use where access is difficult or time is at a premium. Also, physical parameters like temperature, blood pressure and pulse rate are at present very much easier to monitor than chemical parameters like pH, P_{O_2} and P_{CO_2}, which are sometimes more important to the clinician.

The current trend towards miniaturization and improved component reliability and performance will help in removing some of the limitations. Telemetry of physiological signals from within the body is hampered by the bulk of mercury cells, small though it is. Here, as in the case of implanted stimulators like the cardiac pacemaker, there is a need for developing more convenient power sources.

CHAPTER 4

THE NOISY NUCLEUS

The economy of the human body and the elaborate inter-relation of its various components may be described in many ways. The alchemist, the philosopher, the mathematician and the engineer have all made plausible models for this purpose. Current interest in the diagnostic applications of radio-active isotopes reflect the popularity—and the success—of the biochemical and physiological approaches to the study of man. This chapter deals mainly with problems arising from the use of isotopes in biochemical investigation.

All chemical reactions must be identified and studied by indirect means. Biochemistry is a science of recent development—which hardly existed before the beginning of the present century—and one which employs many powerful experimental and intellectual weapons. The biochemist's main concern is to learn about the chemical processes linked with the multitudinous energy transformations by which the body's vital processes are maintained. In this endeavour the biochemist may analyse the raw materials and end products of the metabolic processes, hoping to infer the nature of the intervening reactions. This is not enough; one would learn little about the steam engine by analysing coal, ash and smoke, but the biochemist can study various intermediate stages by sampling blood and other tissues in health and in disease.

To obtain more precise information he has to find some way of investigating chemical processes at the molecular level. Many of the traditional techniques are not suitable—partly because it is difficult to separate one particular reaction from the network of simultaneous chemical changes and partly because the body's chemical equilibrium is too finely balanced to allow substitution or any of the more robust methods available for elucidating structures and transformations in the laboratory.

It is in this situation that radio-active isotopes are peculiarly valuable. Every chemical element exists in one or more (usually several) radio-active varieties or isotopes. They may be made by exposure of the stable element (or a suitable compound) to bombardment by neutrons in a nuclear reactor, or by several other methods which are rather less convenient. The choice of method depends on the isotope which is required, but most of the common applications are based on reactor-made isotopes because of the simplicity and cheapness of the manufacturing process.

To the advantages of low cost and ready availability two further valuable features must be added.

The first is the simplicity and sensitivity of the techniques by which radio-active materials may be recognized and measured. The experimental methods commonly available in the analyst's laboratory will seldom give useful results when the sample contains fewer than 10^{15} atoms of the species under investigation—representing roughly 10^{-7} g. Instruments for the detection of radio-activity will respond to the disintegration of a single atom, and (to be more realistic) will give meaningful information from samples containing 10^6 atoms of the desired species—representing about 10^{-16} g—or even less. Counting equipment of the kind generally available to students, or even to schoolboys, will respond to quantities of material (in radio-active form) far beyond the limits at which traditional methods of analysis are exhausted.

The second major advantage resides in the observation that the chemical and biological properties of a material are in general unchanged when the stable atoms of a particular constituent element are wholly or partly replaced by atoms of a radio-active isotope of the same element. In these circumstances the behaviour of the radio-active constituents may be used as a reliable guide to the behaviour of the corresponding stable element or compound.

Clinical tests

Many methods are available for exploiting the unique properties of radio-active materials in clinical science.

(*a*) In one group of tests the radio-active isotope is used merely as a marker to indicate, for example, the time taken by the blood to pass from one point in the body to another.

(*b*) There are many applications of the dilution technique. Here a small quantity of an appropriate radio-active material is added to some system or compartment of the body—for example, the blood. After an interval to allow mixing, the system under examination is sampled and assayed for radio-activity. Suppose, for example, that a microcurie of tracer is added to a patient's circulation (by injection) and that a 10-ml sample subsequently removed is found to contain $0 \cdot 002 \mu$Ci of activity; simple calculation indicates that the total blood volume of the patient is 5l. It is, of course, necessary to choose a tracer which stays in the circulating blood until the test is completed; many materials disappear very quickly into other tissues. There are other limitations and precautions, but the method is widely useful.

(*c*) The biochemical processes associated with a particular element or compound may be studied by administering a suitable quantity of the material in labelled form and studying its fate in the body. For example, a few microcuries of radio-active iodine may be given (by mouth) to help in assessing the function of the thyroid gland. The subsequent behaviour of the radio-active atoms may be investigated by direct examination of the thyroid gland with a scintillation counter, by radio-active assay of bodily excretions, or by measuring the amount of radio-activity in components of the circulating blood.

(d) A patient may take a small dose of a radio-active material chosen for its ability to concentrate in some particular organ of the body or in a malignant tumour. The subsequent distribution of the isotope is scanned on the intact patient, to build up a picture of the organ concerned and of the biochemical processes occurring in it. Scanning techniques will be reviewed in more detail in another chapter.

(e) The tests already mentioned are usually performed with short-lived isotopes for safety. Useful work can sometimes be done by administering a dose of a long-lived isotope and following its retention and distribution with a whole-body counter. This device offers remarkable sensitivity, though it does not give very detailed information about the location and distribution of the radio-active tracer in the body. Whole-body counting techniques are valuable in relatively slow processes such as bone growth, and in the study of certain blood disorders.

Measurement of radio-activity in absolute units (such as the curie or its subdivisions) is a difficult exercise and is usually attempted only in standardizing laboratories. For clinical use it is always enough to compare the count rates obtained from (a) the original dose, i.e. the dose before administration to the patient—or from an aliquot of this dose, and (b) the patient or the appropriate sample of blood or other material.

It is, of course, necessary that the geometrical relationship between the sample and the counter be the same in both instances. Sometimes one must measure the original dose with a phantom (that is, a dummy patient) in order to reproduce the absorption, scattering and other influences associated with the patient's body.

The main problem is to devise a sensitive counting system by which the radio-activity of the sample can be assayed. Often a quantitative measurement (in count/min) will be enough, but it is sometimes necessary to make qualitative measurements by estimating the energy of the radiation.

Detecting devices

The choice of detector is influenced by the nature of the radiation to be measured.

Virtually every radio-active isotope used in medicine emits beta rays. Many isotopes emit gamma rays as well. When the sample is available in liquid or solid form, beta counting will generally be the most sensitive method. Often, however, it is desired to estimate the amount of radio-activity inside the body, as for example in thyroid function studies. The range of beta rays is seldom more than a couple of centimetres in tissue, so accurate estimation is not possible with detectors outside the body. In these circumstances it is best to count the gamma rays, and, of course, to choose the isotope with this in mind.

In general, the Geiger counter is useful for high-energy beta rays, the liquid scintillation counter for low-energy beta rays and the solid scintillation counter for gamma rays.

The Geiger counter is one of the oldest devices for the detection of ionizing radiations and it still has many applications. Essentially it is a cold-cathode discharge tube triggered by the energy given up when a beta particle (or a gamma ray quantum) is absorbed. A Geiger tube contains two electrodes—a cathode which usually takes the form of a metal cylinder or helix, and an anode in the form of a thin wire along the axis of the cylinder. The tube is filled with a mixture of argon and ethyl alcohol or argon and a halogen gas. The potential difference between the electrodes is maintained at a value somewhat below the break-down potential.

A thin window of mica or glass, fitted to one end of the counter tube, allows the entry of beta radiation from a planchet on which the sample is spread. For the detection of low-energy beta radiation (for example, from ^{3}H and ^{14}C) a demountable windowless counter is sometimes used. Here the sample planchet is inside the counter, through which the filling gas is passed continually.

The Geiger counter is not efficient for the detection of gamma-radiation, but its performance in this respect may be improved by using a cathode coated with lead. Some of the incident gamma-ray quanta will be absorbed in the lead, releasing electrons which are detected by the normal Geiger process.

If the filling gas of a Geiger tube is ionized (for example, by the passage of a beta particle or gamma-ray quantum), the electrons released are accelerated in the high electrical field between the electrodes and themselves cause further ionization. The process is cumulative, resulting in an avalanche of electrons and a corresponding pulse of current in the external circuit.

The Geiger counter is a sensitive device because of the considerable multiplicative effect after the initial ionizing event, but it has no power of discrimination; the output pulse has the same shape and amplitude whatever the energy of the particle or quantum that initiated it.

The efficiency of the Geiger counter is satisfactory for beta rays, reaching 30 per cent or more, but may be only 1 to 2 per cent for gamma rays. Details of the electronic accessories needed for the collection and processing of signals from a Geiger counter will be discussed later.

All methods of radiation detection depend on ionization in one way or another. It follows that a gaseous device like the Geiger counter will generally have low efficiency. Detection by ionization in a solid or a liquid device has two attractions:

(*a*) higher efficiency, especially for gamma rays, since there is clearly a much greater chance of capturing energy from the particle or quantum as it passes through the detector;

(*b*) capturing the whole energy of a gamma-ray quantum and thus eliciting output pulses each proportional in amplitude to the original energy of the responsible quantum: this means that an energy spectrum of the original radiation may be produced, making pulse-height analysis possible.

The solid scintillation counter is a rather complicated arrangement with obvious shortcomings, but is the most widely used device for gamma-ray detection and measurement. It is based on the fluorescence of certain organic and inorganic materials known as phosphors.

Fluorescence was early exploited in the spinthariscope (invented by Crookes) in which the light flashes produced in a layer of zinc sulphide, by an adjacent sample of radio-active material, were counted by eye. The instrument was used successfully by Rutherford and his collaborators in the present century, but was superseded by the Geiger counter. It returned to popularity in the more sophisticated forms developed in a number of laboratories about twenty years ago. The basic improvement was the coupling of the phosphor to a photomultiplier tube (a photo-electric cell with built-in amplifying system) from which electrical signals of adequate proportions could be obtained.

The modern scintillation counter depends on (*a*) the absorption of energy from incident gamma-ray quanta, (*b*) the conversion of this energy (in the process of fluorescence) into flashes of light which cause the cathode of the photomultiplier to emit electrons, and (*c*) the amplification of the initial electron emission (by a factor of about 10^6) to yield an electrical pulse suitable for counting, recording and further treatment.

A scintillation phosphor should have as many as possible of the following properties:

(*a*) high density and atomic number to allow substantial absorption of gamma radiation;

(*b*) good light output;

(*c*) optical transparency;

(*d*) fluorescence with rapid decay so that counting may be fast;

(*e*) low enough refractive index; if it is too high, extraction of light flashes will be difficult because of internal reflexion.

No single material exhibits all of these characteristics (see table) but the requirements for a particular experiment can usually be fulfilled. Sodium iodide, activated by a little thallium, gives good sensitivity, but organic crystals offer a faster decay of the fluorescent light pulses, thus allowing higher counting rates.

Material	Wavelength of maximum emission (Å)	Decay constant (gamma ray excitation) (μs)	Relative pulse height
Inorganic crystals			
NaI (Tl)	4100	0·23	200
CsI (Tl)	4000 to 6000	0·7	90
KI (Tl)	4100	0·24 (56%) : 2·5 (44%)	40
LiI (Eu)	4750	1·2	70
Organic crystals			
Anthracene	4480	0·03	100
Stilbene	4100	0·005	50
Plastic phosphors	Around 4000	0·003 to 0·015	40 to 60
Liquid phosphors	Around 4000	0·002 to 0·008	25 to 80

Liquid phosphors, made by dissolving fluorescent materials in toluene or some other organic solvent, are useful where large-volume detectors are required and also for the detection of low-energy beta rays; the sample of radio-active material can, with certain precautions, be added to the solution, thereby overcoming the difficulty otherwise presented by the very short range of the radiation. The plastic phosphor is analogous to the liquid scintillator, since it is made by polymerization of a solution of fluorescent material in a liquid monomer such as styrene or polyvinyltoluene.

Many of the instrumental difficulties associated with scintillation counting arise from the complicated interaction between gamma-ray quanta and the phosphor. Some of the incident quanta are absorbed so that virtually the whole of the quantum energy is transferred (as kinetic energy) to an electron ejected from an atom of the phosphor in the photo-electric effect. The energy of the electron is, by repeated ionization and excitation, converted into a light pulse, over a time which is short in relation to the luminous decay time of the phosphor. Consequently a single electrical pulse (the photo-peak) is obtained from the output of the photomultiplier.

Unfortunately the absorption in the phosphor of a succession of identical gamma-ray quanta does not produce as the electrical output a train of identical pulses: in other words a sharp line in the gamma-ray spectrum of the radio-active sample is reproduced as a broad peak in the eventual electrical signal.

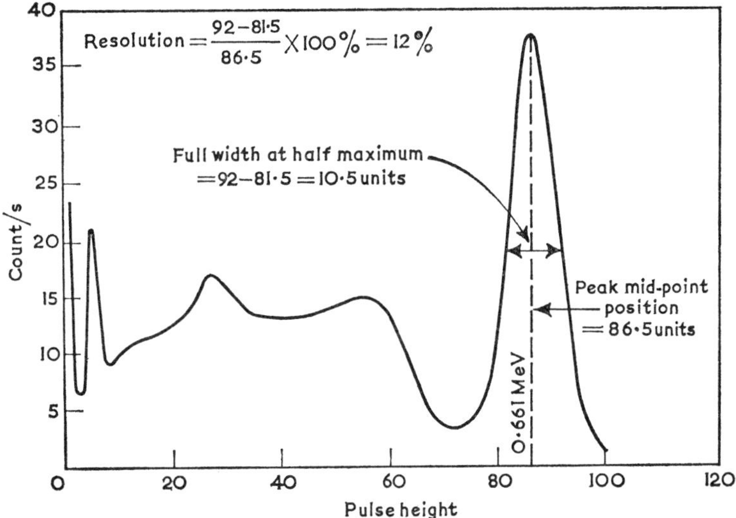

Fig. 15 Typical pulse-height spectrum from a sample of ^{137}Cs. This isotope gives one gamma-ray line of energy 0·661 MeV. (*Courtesy of Harshaw Chemical Co.*)

The main reason for this loss of resolution is to be found in the random fluctuations of electron emission at various stages in the photo-multiplier. The pulse-height spectrum is complicated also because some of the gamma-ray quanta striking the phosphor are absorbed in the Compton effect or in pair production.* In these processes the quantum energy may not be wholly converted into light. For these reasons a flux of quanta all with the same energy will give rise to a train of electrical pulses with widely differing amplitudes, up to a maximum represented by the photo-peak (fig. 15). If, as often,

* The *Compton effect* is the scattering and increase in wavelength of homogeneous X- or gamma-rays by free electrons. The increased wavelength implies a loss of energy by the radiation quantum to the electron. *Pair Production* is the conversion of a photon of radiation into an electron and a positron when it passes through a strong electrical field like that in the neighbourhood of a nucleus or an electron. Here too energy is lost by the radiation.

there are several gamma-ray energies in the radiation emitted by the sample, the resulting spectrum may be quite difficult to analyse and interpret.

Solid-state detectors

The solid-state detector may be regarded as an ionization chamber with semiconducting material instead of gas filling.

In solid-state counters the incident radiation produces electrons and holes in a semiconductor material such as silicon or germanium. The charges so set free are collected by an electric field; sometimes (as in the *pn* junction detector) an internal field is also involved. The average energy expenditure to produce an electron-hole pair in silicon is about 3·5 eV. This is only a tenth of the energy needed to produce an ion pair in a Geiger counter or other device where ionization is the predominant process. The expected advantages of rapid response and good resolution are obtained. Overall efficiency is low for energetic gamma rays (though excellent for charged particles or very soft gamma rays) because of the low atomic number of the materials ($Z = 14$ for silicon) and the small volume of the detectors made by currently-available manufacturing techniques. In certain circumstances (for example, the analysis of mixtures of gamma-emitting isotopes) the excellent resolution outweighs the low sensitivity, but the great potential of solid-state counters has not yet been fully realized in practice.

Liquid scintillation counting

In liquid scintillation counting the sample, the solvent and the scintillator are intimately mixed in a container which is viewed by one or more photomultiplier tubes. The system has two important advantages:

High efficiency. Since the sample material and the scintillator are in the closest contact, there is little chance that a beta particle emitted in radio-active decay will escape from the container without giving up its energy to a molecule of scintillator. It is, of course, not always possible to dispose the photomultiplier tubes so as to collect the whole of the light emitted in the scintillation process, but efficiencies of 50 per cent or more can be obtained, depending on the particular isotope used.

Suitability for low-energy beta radiation. It is a curious dispensation of providence that the four elements hydrogen, carbon, nitrogen and oxygen, which together account for more than 90 per cent of all living matter, are not well provided with radio-active isotopes. ^{3}H (tritium) and ^{14}C are immensely useful in biochemical and clinical investigation, but cannot be detected with reasonable efficiency in simple Geiger or solid scintillation counters; both emit beta radiation of low energy, with no accompanying gamma radiation. The maximum beta-ray energy of tritium is about 18 keV and the corresponding figure for ^{14}C is about 155 keV. Electrons of these energies have very little penetrating power, and would, for example, be heavily absorbed in the window of a conventional Geiger counter or in the light-tight outer sheath of a solid scintillation counter. Self-absorption is also troublesome in a condensed sample (such as a solid layer or a liquid preparation) of the kind which is quite acceptable when dealing with isotopes emitting beta radiation of higher energy. In a liquid scintillation system the beta ray from a disintegrating atom may have to travel a distance of only a few molecular diameters before meeting a molecule of scintillator.

Liquid scintillation counting is proportional, the final electrical pulses having an amplitude distribution corresponding to the energy spectrum of the beta particles delivered by the sample under investigation. This property (shared, of course, with solid scintillation counting) is useful in the double-tracer technique; for example, a complex molecule of biological interest may be labelled at two different places in its structure with tritium and with ^{14}C, allowing metabolic processes to be studied in greater detail than a single tracer would permit.

Complete systems for liquid scintillation counting are available from several manufacturers; they differ mainly in the ingenuity and sophistication of the sample-handling and data-processing facilities which are offered.

Limitations in clinical applications

Techniques used in the medical applications of radio-active isotopes are dominated by the necessity for obtaining an ultimate signal with a maximum content of information, while accepting inevitable—and often severe—limitations on the quantity of radio-activity that can be used or on the overall size of the detector. Some of the factors involved in this optimizing process are as follows.

Background. Every signal obtained from a radiation detector is mixed with random noise contributed by the natural background. Some of the background is attributable to cosmic radiation, some to radio-active materials always naturally in the air, the ground and building materials, and some to the natural radio-activity present at low levels in the glass and metal components of detecting systems. Radio-active isotopes used in various manufacturing processes sometimes find their way into the finished product; contemporary lead, iron and steel are usually contaminated for this reason. The radiation background can be considerably reduced by surrounding the detector with lead; thicknesses of 2 to 4 in (50 to 100 mm) are common. To obtain further improvement it is necessary to use anti-coincidence techniques. Suppose, for example, that an end-window counter is used to detect beta radiation. Some of the background will arise from the absorption (in the counter) of gamma-ray quanta which have penetrated the lead shield. The output pulses which they produce are indistinguishable from those initiated by beta particles from the sample—but there is one way of separating them. Gamma-sensitive Geiger tubes are disposed around the end-window counter to shield it from every aspect; thirty or forty tubes may be required. The output signals from all of the shield tubes are fed to one input terminal of a coincidence circuit, while the output from the end-window counter goes to the other input terminal. The coincidence circuit is designed to register the arrival of a signal from the end-window counter but to reject signals which arrive simultaneously at both input terminals. A background pulse which triggers the end-window counter must have passed first through one of the shield tubes and will therefore not be accepted. But a beta particle from the sample will operate the end-window counter alone (since it cannot penetrate any further) and will be recorded by the coincidence circuit. It is sometimes possible to obtain a considerable degree of shielding for anti-coincidence purposes with a single counter of suitable shape. In one system the shield counter is hemispherical in shape, and near its centre there is a depression into which the end-window sample-counter may be fitted.

Noise. A somewhat similar problem is presented by interference from internal noise in photomultipliers. Thermionic emission from the cathode of a photomultiplier produces a background of random pulses superimposed on the signals derived from the radio-active sample. The interference is particularly troublesome in relation to isotopes emitting low-energy beta radiation, for which the thermal noise pulses are comparable in amplitude with the genuine pulses and therefore not easily distinguished. For this reason the problem is mainly important in liquid scintillation-counting systems. The noise background may be reduced by placing the whole counting system in a refrigerated enclosure at a temperature of about 0°C. Further improvement is achieved by using two photomultipliers in a coincidence circuit (fig. 16). The scintillation pulses will be recorded by both counters but random noise pulses will be rejected since they do not (except by a rare chance) occur simultaneously in both photocathodes.

Electronic accessories

The Geiger counter is a relatively simple device, capable of counting at low rates (up to about 100 count/s), and its operation does not make heavy demands on the electronic designer. The counter gives pulses of uniform amplitude, needing only modest amplification to

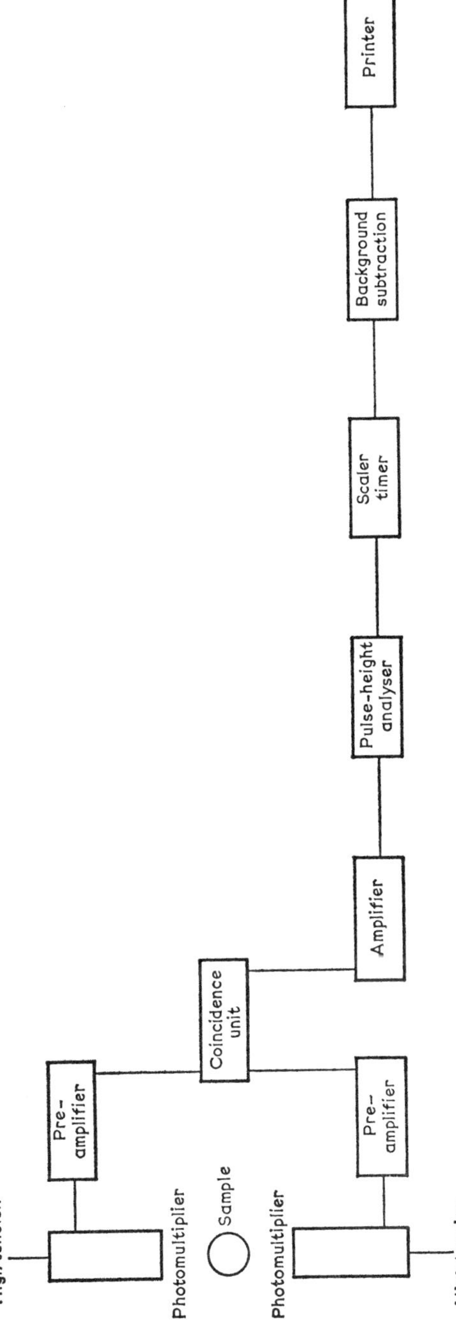

Fig. 16 Schematic arrangement of liquid scintillation counter. Automatic subtraction of background (based on results obtained in a prior counting period) is a useful facility.

operate scaling and counting equipment. Greater ingenuity is needed for scintillation counting, as we shall now explain.

Power supplies. A general-purpose high-tension supply for a Geiger or scintillation counter should have an output adjustable over 0 to 2000 V, with a maximum current of 5 mA. It should offer output stability better than 0·1 per cent against mains variation of 10 per cent. These requirements are not hard to meet.

Amplifiers. It is usually necessary to have a cathode follower unit close to the photomultiplier. The input resistance should be at least 1 MΩ and the input capacitance 1pF. The output impedance will be about 1000 Ω, allowing pulses to be transmitted along several yards (m) of cable without degeneration in rise time. The output pulse from the photomultiplier will have an amplitude of the order of 1 mV and therefore requires considerable amplification before reaching the scaler and counter. A non-overloading amplifier is used; recovery to 1 per cent from a 200$\times$ overload should be achieved in 5 μs. The amplifier output pulse should have an amplitude proportional to the energy lost in the original ionizing event in the phosphor. This means that the output pulse amplitude should be proportional to the time integral of the current pulse from the photomultiplier. The output pulse usually has an amplitude of about 10 V, a rise time of about 0·2 μs and a duration of the order of 1 μs.

Pulse-height analysis. A simple technique is to use discriminator circuits, which can be arranged to pass only the pulses which are of above—or below—a specified amplitude. A solid scintillation counter (for high-energy gamma rays) always includes a discriminator to eliminate the low-energy pulses resulting from photomultiplier noise. Two discriminators in series can be arranged to form a 'window' which, when swept through the energy range, will produce a spectrum of the radiation under investigation. A single-channel pulse-height analyser of this kind requires considerable time to give a detailed spectrum, in which the energy range may be divided into at least a hundred channels. The method is clearly unsuitable for short-lived activities, where the counting rate will change between the beginning and end of the sweep. In the multi-channel analysers now commonly used, counting proceeds simultaneously (rather than sequentially) in a hundred or more channels. Early designs involved an array of single-channel analysers, each with its own display facility. It is difficult to obtain complete coverage of the energy range without overlap between adjacent channels. Errors are also introduced by drift or other instability in individual channels. The modern multi-channel analyser uses different methods. Each incoming pulse is converted from an analogue into a digital quantity; the number generated in this way is stored at an appropriate address in a magnetic memory which is afterwards scanned to reproduce the complete spectrum. The conversion may be achieved in a number of ways. The incoming pulse may, for example, be stretched to give a continuous signal of the same amplitude. A ramp pulse is generated separately, starting from zero amplitude and increasing linearly with time. An oscillator or pulse generator, turned on at the same instant as the ramp pulse, measures (digitally) the time taken for the ramp pulse to reach the same amplitude as the signal. The amplitude of the signal pulse is thus converted into a digital equivalent, which represents the address of one section in the analyser memory. The content (binary) of the appropriate section is then increased by unity. The pulse-height spectrum is obtained, when required, by scanning the memory and transferring its contents to an oscillograph screen, $X–Y$ recorder or print-out device.

Scaling, counting and timing units. When it is desired to investigate the total counting rate (rather than the pulse-height spectrum) relatively simple electronic devices may be used; the problem of determining and displaying total counts or counting rates is, of course, familiar in many industrial and scientific situations. Dekatron tubes, serving both to count and to display, are still widely used; their maximum counting rate (about 20 000 count/s) is enough for most clinical and biological investigations. More recently designed equipment uses transistors for counting and cold-cathode tubes for display, offering higher counting rates (up to 1 MHz) and higher storage capacity. At high counting rates a buffer store is useful in eliminating loss of counts during the interval required for transfer to the display system. When many samples have to be counted (as is common in clinical investigations) an automatic sample-changer is useful. This mechanical device present the samples to the counter in sequence; the counter may be adjusted to study each sample for a pre-set time or a pre-set number of counts before printing out the numerical findings. With these facilities the counting system may be left unattended for long periods. The use of a counting ratemeter is often convenient, despite the inevitable loss of information content in comparison with digital recording. Input pulses are adjusted to a uniform amplitude and shape before passing through a diode pump into a CR circuit across which a voltage-measuring device is connected. When equilibrium conditions are reached the potential difference across the condenser is proportional to the rate of arrival of pulses. At a constant counting rate the time taken to reach equilibrium is determined by the time constant, CR, which also regulates the response of the device to the fluctuating counting rates more often encountered in practice.

Medical applications

In Britain, isotope techniques are applied mainly in large central hospitals where equipment is more easily obtained and where scientific and technical advice is more readily available. The demand from peripheral hospitals for suitable facilities is small, mainly because the range of simple and useful routine tests is surprisingly limited.

In general, the results of isotope tests alone do not provide sufficient information for conclusive diagnosis. Often numbers of laboratory tests demanding skilful interpretation are required to provide adequate confirmation. It is probably fortunate, therefore, that the scarce available resources are concentrated at central hospitals.

In several relatively simple tests useful information can be obtained by monitoring the accumulation or clearance of molecules labelled with gamma emitters using a detector outside the body and collimated to view a single organ.

Tracer tests

For example, a great deal of knowledge regarding thyroid function can be acquired by measuring the rate of uptake in the thyroid of a dose of ^{131}I given orally. Normally the activity is monitored using a sodium iodide crystal, typically 5 cm in diameter by 3 cm thick, about 20 cm from the gland. A counting period of less than 1 min generally provides excellent statistical accuracy. This simple test will often confirm clinical evidence, but more complex tests using isotopes are necessary in difficult cases.

In haematology some information regarding iron metabolism can be deduced by monitoring the behaviour of an injected dose of ^{59}Fe over the heart, spleen, liver and sacrum (a flat bone at the base of the spine). The activity from the heart essentially measures the relative level of ^{59}Fe in the blood. In more complex ways the activity from the sacrum reflects the rate of incorporation of iron into red cells and the activities from the spleen and liver are related to the breakdown of old red cells. In this test the metabolic processes are relatively slow and the investigation will extend over several days. Each site can be monitored for several minutes at a time with good statistical accuracy.

Radio-active inert gases such as ^{133}Xe and ^{85}Kr are finding wide application in the determination of organ blood flow and in the study of heart or lung function. One of their attractive properties is that they diffuse very rapidly into the lungs from the blood stream, so that problems associated with the recirculation of isotopes are minimized. This property forms the basis of a method of studying lung function.

A relatively large dose of ^{133}Xe is injected into a vein and the levels of activity over selected sites on the chest are monitored using an array of sodium iodide scintillation detectors. Over sites where lung function is normal there will be an almost immediate response owing to the rapid diffusion of xenon into the lungs. Over other areas the response will be considerably reduced.

Blood flow in the brain can be determined by monitoring the clearance of ^{133}Xe from regions selected by collimation of a scintillation detector outside the skull. The xenon dissolved in saline is introduced *via* the artery supplying the brain. In the capillaries the gas diffuses rapidly into the surrounding tissues. When injection ceases the normal circulation flushes out the inert tracer, the rate of removal being very closely related to blood flow. The clearance is monitored for approximately 10 min and the data are usually presented on a potentiometric pen recorder driven by a counting rate-meter.

In more sophisticated systems several sites are studied simultaneously. In such cases a multichannel digital tape recorder and a digital ratemeter provide more convenient data processing facilities.

The range of application of external counting techniques is clearly limited and most of the routine studies involve sample counting. In these tests elaborate biochemical separations are possible, so the information content of a single test is often considerably enhanced.

In haematology the behaviour of red cells can be studied by following the progress of red cells labelled with ^{51}Cr. Samples of blood are removed at intervals over several weeks and the red cells counted in a well-type NaI crystal detector. Red cell survival rates can easily be calculated after correcting for radio-active decay.

Almost all metabolic processes can now be studied with the aid of labelled compounds. Unfortunately, the choice of labelling elements is often confined to low-energy beta-emitters such as ^{3}H, ^{14}C and ^{35}S. In these cases *in vivo* measurements are virtually impossible and sample counting using liquid scintillation counters or end-window gas counters is required.

Total body water can be determined by a dilution technique involving the counting of tritiated water* in a liquid scintillation counter.

Information regarding the metabolism of calcium and strontium in bone can be gained indirectly by measuring the variation in the levels of ^{45}Ca (a beta emitter) or ^{85}Sr (a gamma emitter) in urine and blood over a period of time. Skilful interpretation of the data is required.

The hopes which accompanied the arrival of radio-active isotopes in the clinical realm have not been fulfilled. It was, for example, widely predicted that the new materials would be useful in the diagnosis and—more especially—the treatment of cancer. It has, however, proved impossible (with rare exceptions) to obtain in a tumour a

* Water labelled with tritium.

sufficient concentration of any radio-active material (taken by mouth or by injection) to give a useful therapeutic effect.

In diagnostic work and in the unravelling of physiological processes radio-active isotopes have contributed to substantial achievements by professional biochemists as well as by clinical research workers. Though isotope techniques are now concentrated in well-equipped centres in Britain, their use is more widely diffused in countries such as the United States, where the private practitioner has an appreciable share in the work. Some techniques will probably be absorbed into the routine of the British hospital laboratory. Here it is important to have simple and reliable instruments; the developments reviewed in this chapter offer a good foundation for future expansion of isotope studies in clinical science and technology.

CHAPTER 5

THE INNER EYE

In many respects the body may be regarded as a highly complex mechanical and chemical system. Unfortunately, unlike man-made machines, it cannot be taken apart and examined when malfunction is suspected. One of the great challenges in medicine has therefore been to devise, for the investigation of internal organs, techniques that interfere as little as possible with the healthy functioning of the body.

There are several approaches to this problem. One that has met with considerable success has been the direct examination of organs using instruments external to the body. To date, this method has required that the instruments receive information concerning the organ either in the form of electrical energy arising within the organ or in the form of electromagnetic radiation or ultrasound reflected from or transmitted through the organ. In practice, the useful techniques involve X-radiation, radio-active isotopes, ultrasonics and infra-red radiation. Radiography—undoubtedly the best known and most commonly used method—has been the most successful.

Techniques involving radio-active isotopes can be quite powerful both in the delineation of bodily organs (radio-isotope scanning) and in the assessment of organ function. The successful application of ultrasonics in medicine is more difficult than in other fields largely because of the highly complex anatomical structure of the body. However, much progress has been made, and the technique is likely to find wider application in the future. The diagnosis of disease by infra-red detection methods (thermography) is in its infancy and has not been used clinically to any great extent.

Radiography

Since the discovery of X-rays by Röntgen in 1895, radiographic techniques have been applied extensively in medicine. At present, it has been estimated, they are used in over 20 per cent of all diagnosis. In recent years the introduction of image intensifiers and combinations of these with closed-circuit television systems has extended the range of routine applications to include the study of dynamic (as well as static) systems. Many of these recent applications are in the study of organ function. Earlier techniques were directed mainly towards the study of organ form.

Production of X-rays

X-rays are always produced when high-energy electrons strike any material. In a typical X-ray tube (fig. 17) electrons, from a heated filament in the cathode, are accelerated in an intense field produced by an applied voltage of the order of 100 kV before striking a suitable target (usually tungsten) and producing a beam of X-rays. This beam is extracted through a thin window in the wall of an evacuated tube and is collimated, using an aperture of variable dimensions in a lead diaphragm.

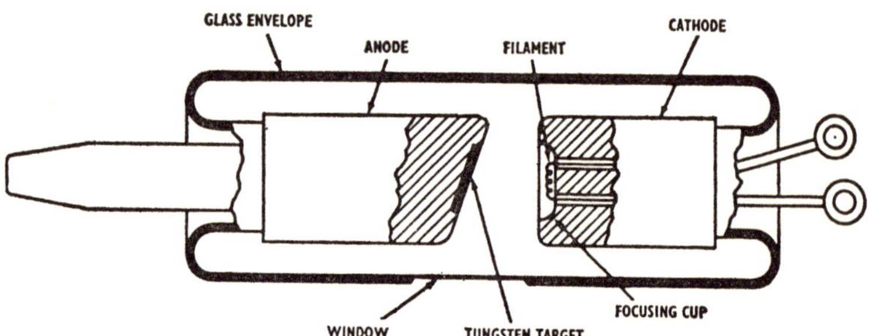

Fig. 17 Diagram of stationary-anode X-ray tube showing relation of anode and cathode. (*Courtesy of Kodak Ltd.*)

X-ray tubes

Most of the energy of the electron beam is converted into heat in the target. Removal of this heat is one of the major considerations in the design and performance of X-ray tubes. In some tubes the capacity to withstand heat is increased by using an anode, in the form of a disk, that rotates rapidly about an axis parallel to the incident electron beam which is directed towards the edge of the disk. In this way the heat is generated round the edge of the target rather than at a small spot, as in tubes with stationary anodes.

X-ray spectra

The spectrum of the energies of the X-rays produced from the tube depends on the energy of the incident electron beam, the nature of the target and the design of the beam exit window. Fig. 18 shows the spectrum obtained from a tungsten target when a voltage of 100 kV is applied.

X-rays are produced by high-energy electrons in two processes, both of which occur in the case shown. In the broad continuous part of the spectrum they are produced when the incident electrons are decelerated in the electric fields surrounding the tungsten nuclei. These radiations are referred to as bremsstrahlung.

The maximum energy of bremsstrahlung is the same as the peak energy of the incident electrons. The minimum energy is zero, but in practice most of the low-energy radiation is absorbed in the beam exit window and in filters introduced for that purpose.

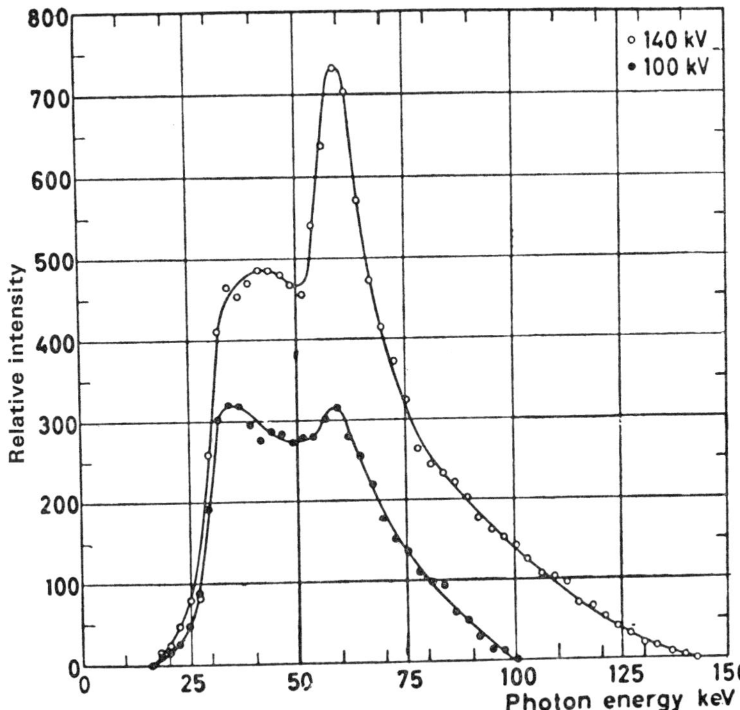

Fig. 18 Spectrum of X-rays from tungsten target. (Based on data collected by G. Hettinger and N. Starfelt, *Acta Radiologica*, Vol. 50, 381 (1958).)

The sharp peaks in the spectrum (characteristic radiation) result from X-rays produced when incident electrons remove orbital electrons from the tungsten atoms. The peaks can only occur when the energy of the incident electrons exceeds the binding energies of the electrons in the orbits.

The spectrum of X-ray energies produced (sometimes described as the *beam quality*) can be controlled by the tube operating voltage and to a certain extent by the nature of the filters used.

Basic techniques

In all diagnostic applications, the organ under study is interposed between the X-ray tube and a suitable detector, such as a photographic film, fluorescent screen or image intensifier, on which an image of the transmitted beam is formed. The image is always magnified by a factor determined by the tube-object and object-detector distances.

In static studies the best definition is achieved using photographic film. Blurring of the image owing to patient movement is minimized by using a high exposure rate for a very short time (of the order of 1/10 s). The tube current is usually of the order of 100 to 300 mA.

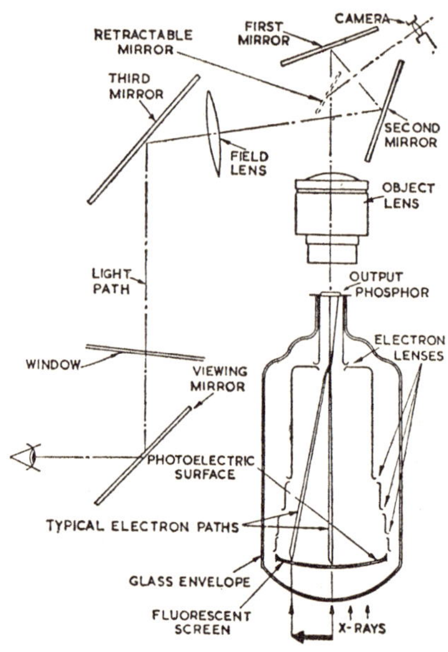

Fig. 19 A typical image intensifier tube

In many applications the transmitted X-ray beam is converted into a visible image in a fluoroscopic screen, generally of zinc sulphide with small amounts of cadmium added. The intensity of light produced at a point in the screen depends on the intensity of the incident X-rays. This system is inherently inefficient; consequently the dose of X-rays has to be increased above that necessary using film only, to produce a visible image. In some circumstances the increase can be justified. For example, in mass radiography the effort and expense involved in developing and examining hundreds of thousands of life-size X-ray film of chests would be prohibitive, whereas satisfactory results can be achieved by using fluoroscopic screens and recording the pictures on rolls of 70-mm film which can be handled comparatively easily. In this case the radiation dose may be increased by a factor of approximately 5.

The main reason for the poor efficiency of simple systems using fluoroscopic screens is that the light produced by incident X-rays is emitted in all directions and therefore only a small fraction will enter the eye of an observer.

Image intensifier systems

The disadvantage is overcome to a large extent using the image intensifier tube; a simple version is illustrated in fig. 19. The back surface of a fluorescent screen is covered with a thin layer of photo-electric material which converts the photons from the screen into electrons. These are accelerated in the evacuated enclosure and focused, using a series of electron lenses, on to a second, much smaller, fluorescent screen to produce an intensified image. The brightness of the final image is increased by a factor of several thousands, partly owing to a diminution in the area of the second screen (typically by a factor of approximately a hundred) and partly to an increase in the number of visible photons produced by the incident high-energy electrons.

The great advantage of image intensifiers is that they readily allow dynamic processes to be studied using X-rays. For example, by exposing the patient to a continuous beam of X-rays, a cardiologist can follow continuously on an image intensifier screen the passage of a thin tube (of a material that absorbs X-rays) through a vein or an artery into the heart.

Cardiac catheterization is only one of a number of important applications of image intensifiers in diagnostic radiology.

Dynamic processes can also be studied using the technique of cinefluorography, in which the X-ray beam is pulsed and the image on the intensifier screen is photographed, using a camera with a shutter that opens in synchronism with the beam pulses. Frame rates of the order of twenty a second are typical.

Closed-circuit television systems

The X-ray dose rates required for diagnostic studies can be reduced by using closed-circuit television systems to display the outputs of the image intensifiers. Various arrangements of fluorescent screens, image intensifiers and television camera tubes are possible. Fig. 20 shows one of these. In this arrangement the intensified image on the screen of the image amplifier is viewed using an image orthicon (a high-sensitivity television camera tube) and the final image displayed on the television screen.

Closed-circuit television has many important applications in radiography. For example, an X-ray picture showing only the blood vessels in an organ can be obtained by subtracting the output of one camera (viewing an X-ray picture of the organ) from the output of a

C

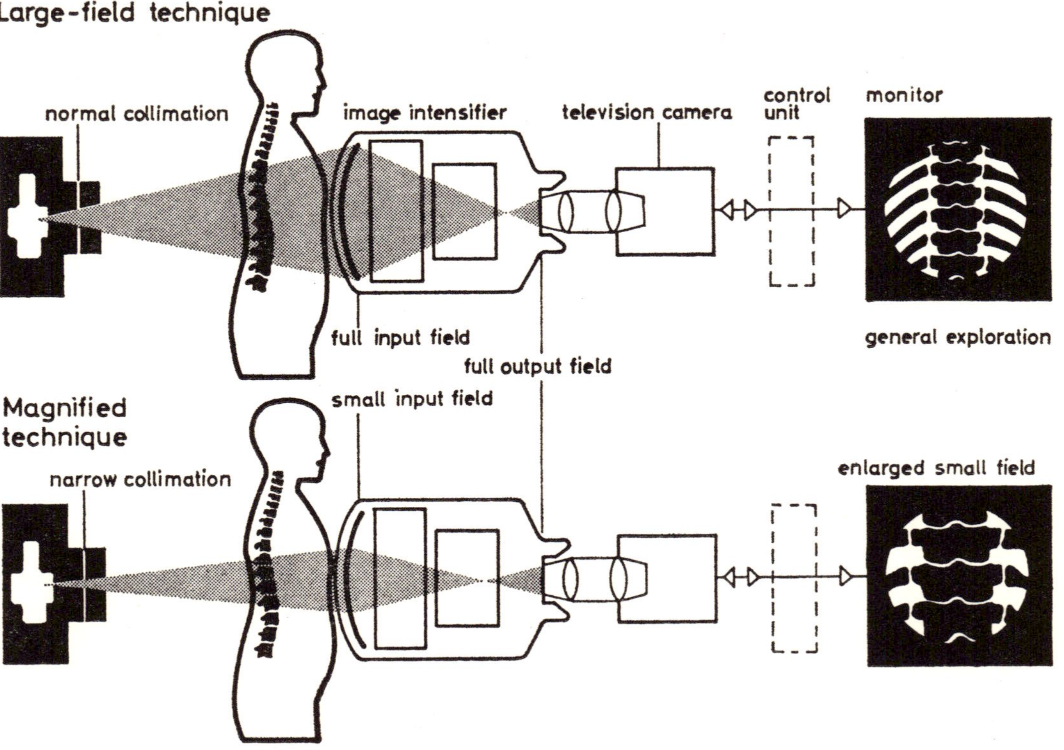

Fig. 20 Image intensifier, television camera and monitor. (*Courtesy of Siemens.*)

second camera, simultaneously viewing a second picture of the organ, obtained after a substance, opaque to X-rays, had been injected into the blood passing through the organ. All features, apart from the radio-opaque substance in the blood vessels, are common to both pictures and are therefore eliminated.

Another important advantage of television systems is that the information can be stored using video tape recorders and can be replayed under various conditions of brightness and contrast.

Stereo-radiography

One difficulty with normal X-ray films is that no impression of depth can be obtained. This can be a serious drawback when complex anatomical features are present. However, the difficulty can be overcome using stereo-radiographic techniques. In the simplest, two X-ray pictures of an organ are taken from positions corresponding to the left and right eyes and the developed films are viewed simultaneously, one by the left eye and the other by the right eye, using a simple optical arrangement. Providing the observer has good binocular vision, depth perception is possible.

This simple idea can be extended to allow dynamic processes to be followed stereoscopically using twin X-ray tubes, twin-pulsed image orthicons viewing an image intensifier screen alternately, twin television sets, and, as before, an optical arrangement for viewing the two sets simultaneously.

Radio-isotope scanning

Radio-isotope scanning is a diagnostic procedure which is being used more extensively as new radio-active tracers become available and scanning equipment improves. The procedure has already been applied successfully to many organs, including the thyroid gland, kidneys, pancreas, heart, spleen, liver, lungs and brain.

The technique involves the study of the distribution of a tracer, introduced into the body by intravenous injection, and known to be selectively taken up by the organ. In this way abnormalities in form or function can often be revealed. A map of the distribution can in general be constructed using either of two techniques.

Moving detector systems

The first mapping technique, developed in the early 1950s, still predominates. It involves scanning the field with an external collimated detector that responds only to radiation arising from a small volume directly beneath it. An analogue of the concentration pattern is formed either on a fixed paper, (by a marker moving in synchronism with the detector) or on a fixed photographic film by a moving

c2

intermittent light source. The density on the paper or the blackening on the developed film is often arranged to be proportional to the concentration of tracer. The results are good but the process is slow, as the picture has to be built up line by line.

The detector used is a sodium iodide crystal, frequently 7·5 cm in diameter and 2·5 cm thick, and sometimes as large as 13 cm in diameter and 5 cm thick. Stray radiation is prevented from reaching the crystal by a thick lead shield which surrounds it. The field of view of the detector is defined by a collimator which consists of a series of converging tapered holes drilled through the lead and focused at a spot some 75 to 150 mm from the face of the shield. Radiation arising at the focus has the best chance of being detected; the probability of detection falls rapidly with increasing distance from the focus. The precise source of the detected radiation is determined from the instantaneous position of the detector collimator assembly, not from the point of incidence of radiation on the crystal.

The crystal is viewed by a photomultiplier tube with the electronic auxiliary equipment discussed in chapter 4. A discriminator rejects thermal noise and reduces the confusion due to scattered radiation, which is always less energetic than radiation direct from the source.

Typical counting rates are 10 to 50/s, depending on the investigation, although rates of less than this are the rule for some organs, i.e. the brain.

At low counting rates the mechanical marker is set to respond to each pulse; at high rates a variable reduction factor is used to allow the marker to respond and to maintain the visible separation of the marks. In some commercial scanners a multi-colour print-out is provided. Here the colour of the printer is related to the counting rate over the area.

Maps of tracer distribution are displayed on developed films superimposed on X-ray outlines of the skull obtained using standard procedures.

One disadvantage of the method is that it is slow, some 20 or 30 min being required for a single picture. This has, however, been improved in a new instrument which has ten adjacent detectors scanning the field. Each detector is capable of counting at the same rate as a single crystal system so that the assembly can count ten times as fast as a conventional scanner. The image being produced can be displayed on a television screen and a permanent record of the scan can be obtained from an oscilloscope using a Polaroid camera.

Moving detector systems have the disadvantage that the whole field cannot be viewed simultaneously and therefore their application is confined to relatively slow dynamic processes. To date this has not been a serious limitation in routine investigations but it does reduce the usefulness of the instrument in serial studies and in applications using short-lived isotopes.

Stationary detector systems

An entirely different approach is to use a stationary instrument which can simultaneously detect radiation from all parts of the organ without mechanical scanning. For historical rather than logical reasons such instruments are also referred to as scanners.

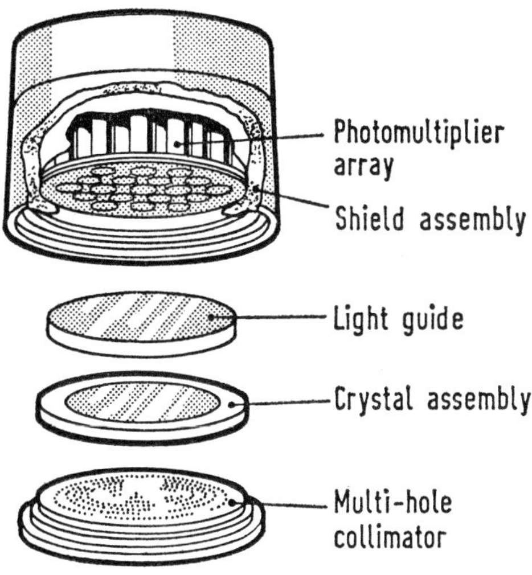

Fig. 21 Exploded diagram of detector-collimator assembly of 11 in (280 mm) gamma camera. (*Courtesy of Nuclear Enterprises (G.B.) Ltd.*).

Gamma cameras

Probably the most advanced and certainly the most commonly used of such scanners is the gamma camera (fig. 21). There are two types, one with a single pin-hole and the other with a large number of parallel apertures.

In principle the pin-hole gamma camera is similar to an ordinary pin-hole camera. In both cases there is inversion of the image, which, in the gamma camera, is displayed on an oscilloscope screen.

The detector is a large sodium iodide crystal, 13 to 28 cm in diameter and up to 2·5 cm thick. The precise point at which the gamma ray strikes the crystal indicates the source of radiation in the organ. Simultaneous signals from all of the tubes are processed to locate the incident gamma ray (fig. 22). Clearly, the closer a particular tube is to that point, the larger will be the signal in that channel.

In most instruments the image is displayed on an oscilloscope

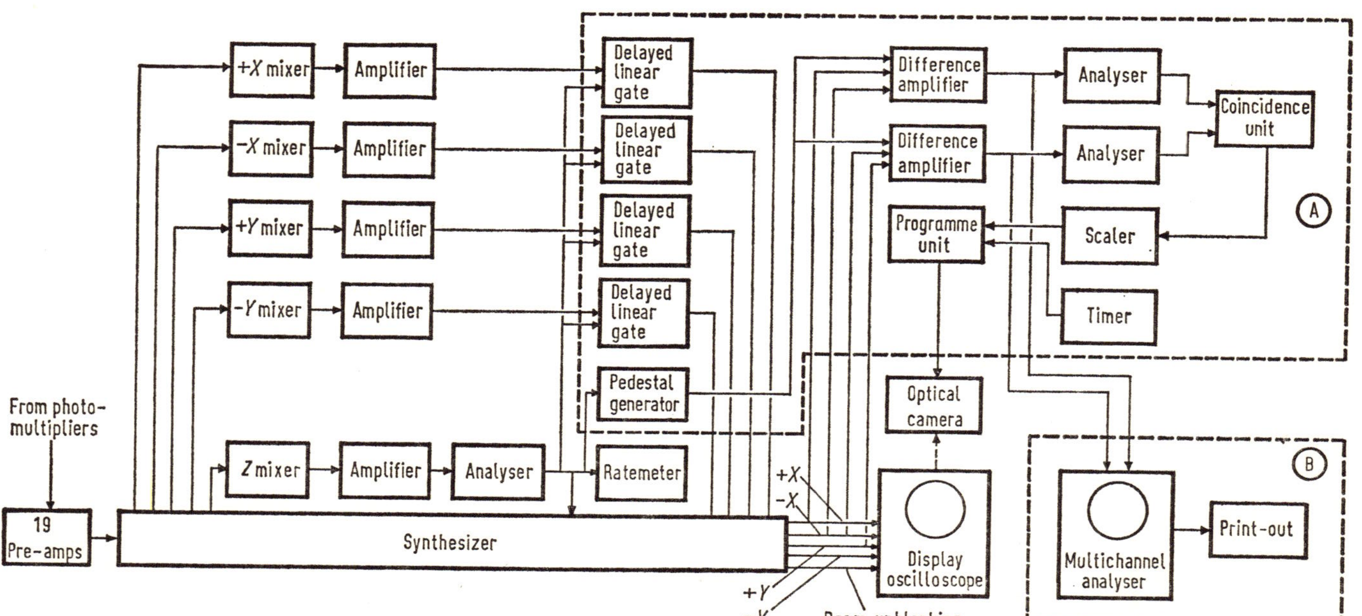

Fig. 22 Block diagram of electronic circuits of gamma camera shown in Fig. 21.

screen. Appropriate fractions of the photomultiplier signal are added and used to control the voltages on the deflexion plates of the cathode-ray tube. The electron beam is switched on only when the combined signals fall within a preselected band corresponding to the photo-peak. In the early instruments only a small fraction of the photo-peak was used because the electronic circuits were not sufficiently developed to cope satisfactorily with the spectrum of signals (discussed in chapter 4) obtained from mono-energetic radiation. However, the introduction of ratio circuits, which essentially modify all of the simultaneous signals from the photomultiplier tubes by a factor that is varied in such a way that the combined signal is always constant, allows the whole of the photo-peak to be used.

Another method of achieving a similar result is to pass the signals from the photomultiplier tubes through amplifiers with logarithmic responses before using them to generate the deflexion signals. The use of logarithmic amplifiers, it is claimed, also helps to overcome one of the major disadvantages in the early instruments—the non-uniformity of response over the field. However, this problem is not likely to be completely solved just by improvements in the electronic circuitry as the irregularity is due also to crystal imperfections and light-collection difficulties.

Another problem with gamma cameras is that the light from each scintillation is shared between all of the photomultipliers so that the random fluctuations in the signals from them will be much larger than the corresponding fluctuations in the signals from a single photo-multiplier system. This is not a serious problem when the incident radiation is of high energy, but at low energy the random fluctuations produce significant variations in the positioning signals.

The pin-hole gamma camera is best suited to the scanning of thin, flat objects as there is an inherent lack of spatial resolution. This uncertainty is removed with the multi-aperture camera, which has a collimator consisting of a large array of narrow, parallel holes normal to the surface of the crystal.

The gamma camera is superior to conventional scanners in that its sensitivity is an order of magnitude higher and it can be used to visualize a whole organ at one time. Dynamic studies of the functioning of organs are possible using exposure times of the order of several seconds. One disadvantage is that the positional resolution is of the order of a centimetre, which is relatively poor. Another disadvantage, mentioned earlier, is the lack of uniformity over the field.

The digital auto-fluoroscope

In principle, the problem of non-uniformity is overcome in the digital auto-fluoroscope (fig. 23), a device which has a detector that consists typically of a 14×21 cm rectangular array of 294 sodium

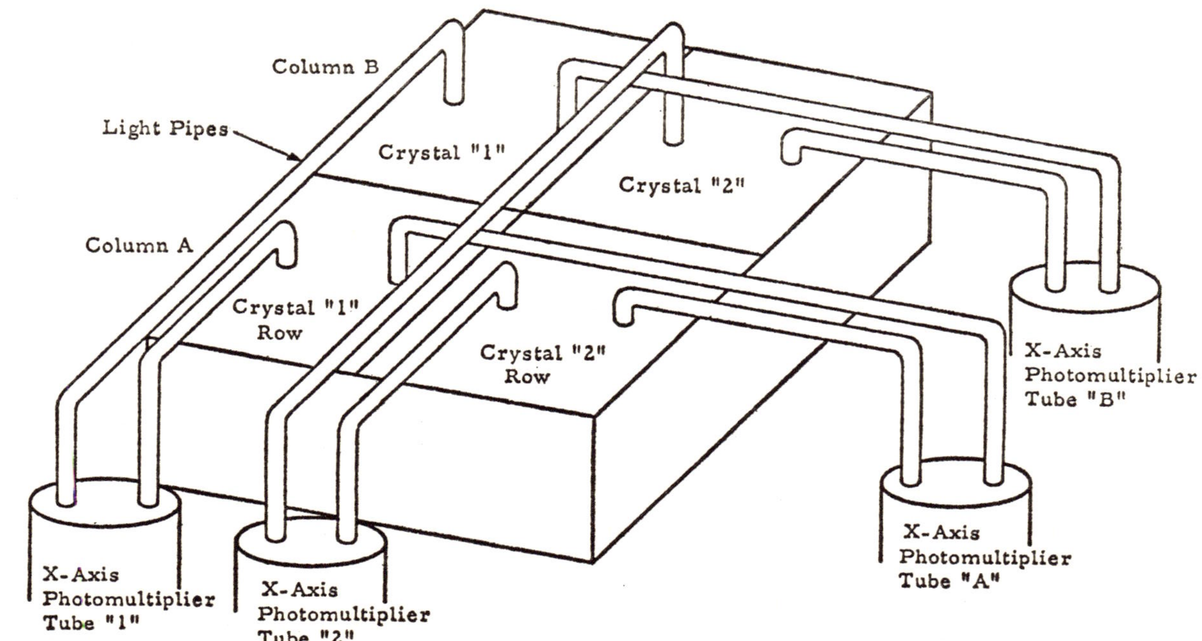

Fig. 23 Principle of arrangement of crystals, light pipes and photomultipliers in the Digital Auto-fluorscope. (*Courtesy of Baird Atomic.*)

iodide crystals, 1 cm square in cross section and 3·8 cm thick. Each crystal is exposed to radiation from the organ via a single hole in a multi-grid collimator. Two light pipes lead from each crystal to an array of photomultiplier tubes. The light pipes and the photo-multiplier tubes are arranged so that each row and each column are viewed by single photo-multiplier tubes. In this way the co-ordinates of a scintillation can be determined.

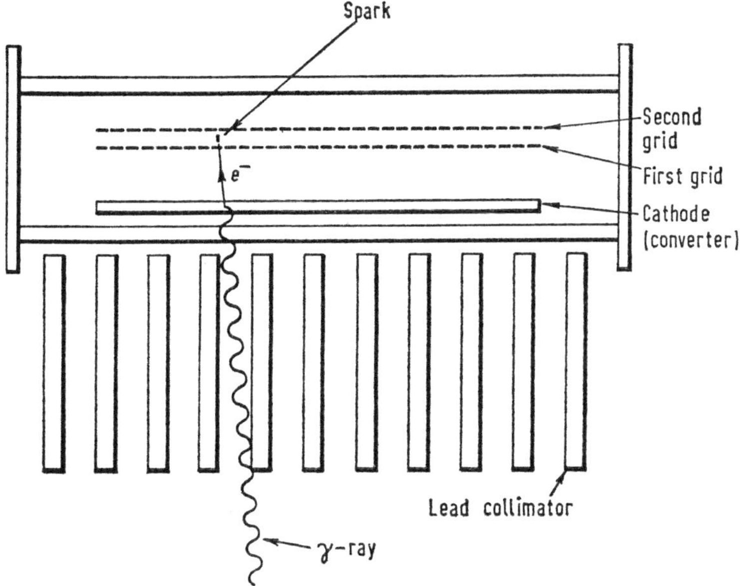

Fig. 24 Diagram of spark chamber.

The instrument has many of the advantages of the gamma camera. It can view a relatively large field at one time, it has high sensitivity—partly because thick crystals with good stopping power can be used and partly because the whole photo-peak, and indeed a large fraction of the Compton continuum, can be accepted without the use of complicated electronic circuitry. Spatial resolution can, however, be no less than the dimension of the individual crystals. Digital information can be readily extracted owing to the simplicity of the method of data processing. An advantage which the instrument has over the gamma camera (in addition to uniformity of response over the field) is that it can cope with significantly higher count rates.

The relatively poor resolution can be a major disadvantage in tumour localization, which is one of the important applications of radio-isotope scanning. Until this is improved the instrument is best suited to the quantitative dynamic study of organ function.

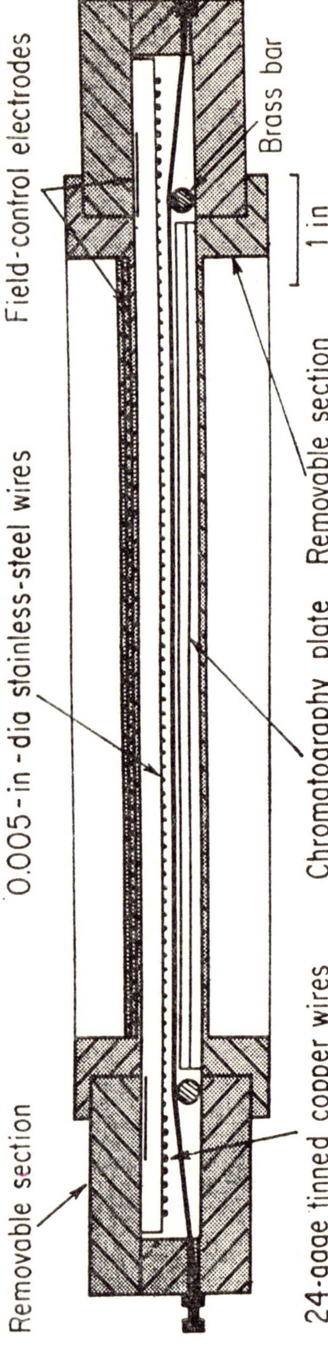

Fig. 25 Cross-section of cross-wired spark chamber. (B. R. Pullan, R. Howard and B. J. Perry, *Nucleonics*, Vol. 24, No. 7, p. 72.) (*Courtesy of McGraw-Hill Inc.*)

Self-triggered spark chambers

Much of the high cost of the stationary detector systems just discussed arises from the complicated electronic arrangements required to determine the point of interaction of the incident radiation and to represent that point on the image. At present only an instrument that uses a self-triggered spark chamber as detector can do this at low cost. Two kinds of spark chamber are available. The first (fig. 24) is filled with xenon at, or slightly above, atmospheric pressure. A fraction of the incident radiation interacts in the aluminium cathode or in the 2-cm gap between anode and grid to produce photo-electrons which are accelerated in a field of 5000 V/cm to the grid. A Townsend avalanche is produced in the much more intense field of 18 000 V/cm in the 4-mm gap between the grid and anode, and this is followed by a spark. The sparks are photographed using a camera with open shutter.

The sensitivity depends mainly on the conversion efficiency of the xenon. With ^{197}Hg (80 keV) the efficiency is approximately 7 per cent. At higher energies sensitivity deteriorates and further problems arise owing to the relative increase in sensitivity to radiation scattered in the organ and in the walls of the collimator (which is always of lower energy). One other disadvantage is that energy discrimination is not possible, but this may not be serious. The recovery time of the chamber limits the sparking rate to a hundred sparks a second but prospects are that this will be improved in future models by using hydrogen thyratrons or ignitrons, triggered by the sparks, to quench the discharges. The instrument is cheap and is likely to find a place in routine diagnosis.

The second kind of chamber (fig. 25) has two parallel electrodes consisting of sets of wires stretched at right-angles to one another and separated by a 2·5-mm gap. A p.d. of 5000 V is applied between the electrodes, and the chamber is continuously flushed with a mixture of argon and methane at atmospheric pressure. Incident radiation is absorbed mainly in an aluminium converter and not in the gas in the chamber. The efficiency of this kind of chamber is low, but a reasonable overall efficiency can be achieved by using a number of chambers arranged in a stack. The arrangement of wires on the electrodes allow the co-ordinates of each spark to be determined relatively simply.

Image intensifier cameras

Interesting new stationary-detector scanning devices, that use image intensifiers instead of sodium iodide photomultiplier assemblies, are under active development (fig. 26). Simple versions use conventional X-ray image amplifiers of the kind used in diagnostic radiology. Incoming gamma rays that have passed through the holes of the collimator are converted in a thin phosphor into light which in turn produces electrons. These are accelerated before striking a suitable phosphor to give an intensified image of the original pattern. Typical light gains are of the order of 5000. One disadvantage of the instruments is that their efficiency is low for detecting radiation of the energy (100 to 300 keV) of most of the isotopes used clinically.

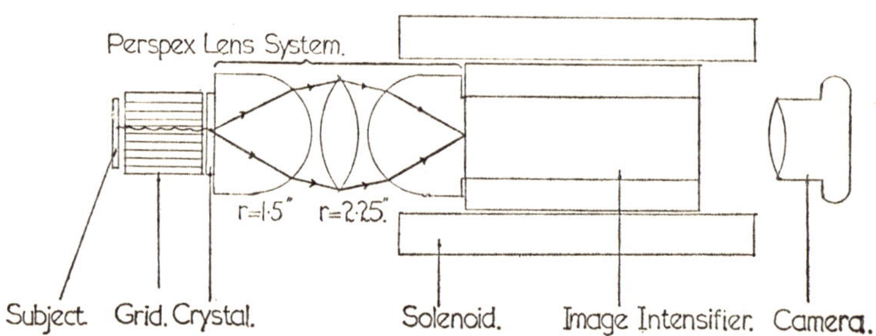

Fig. 26 Image intensifier scanning device with parallel-holed lead collimator, CsI (Tl) crystal, perspex lens system, image intensifier and Polaroid camera. (R. J. Wilks and J. R. Mallard, *Physics in Medicine and Biology*, Vol. 12, No. 2, p. 252.) (*Courtesy of Taylor and Francis Ltd.*)

Recent versions have been built with sodium iodide or caesium iodide crystals, 2 to 5 mm thick, in contact with the photocathode of the image amplifier. Multi-stage amplifiers having light gains of approximately 5×10^5 are used, and the images are photographed with Polaroid cameras.

These instruments should eventually offer sensitivity comparable with that of the gamma camera, spatial resolution down to 1 mm and good uniformity of response over the field. Energy levels will be discriminated by pulsing the image amplifier with a signal derived from a photomultiplier tube coupled to the sodium iodide crystal or from one of the stages of the image amplifier.

It is clear that there is considerable scope for development of scanning techniques but it is important that the cost of the instruments should be kept low; otherwise radio-isotope scanning will never be used extensively in routine diagnosis. The challenge is to produce relatively cheap equipment that can make the distribution of tracer in an organ visible in a matter of seconds, that has spatial resolution of the order of a few millimetres, and that can discriminate against radiation that has energy outside a narrow band.

Studies of organ function using radio-isotopes

In most routine investigations using radio-isotope scanners, the relevant information is obtained from a study of the tracer distribution in the organ at a preselected time. There are several clinical tests, however, in which the important consideration is not the distribution of the tracer but rather the rate at which the tracer accumulates in and is cleared from the organ. In these tests the whole organ or large parts of the organ are viewed using one or several stationary collimated detectors. The behaviour of the tracer is followed in some cases for up to half an hour and in others at fixed times over a period of several days. These kinds of test have been used successfully for many years to study the functions of organs such as the kidneys, thyroid gland and lungs. Essentially the same kind of equipment is used for all of the tests but different tracers are required. Only the test of kidney function (renography) will be described in detail here as the general principles involved apply to all of the tests.

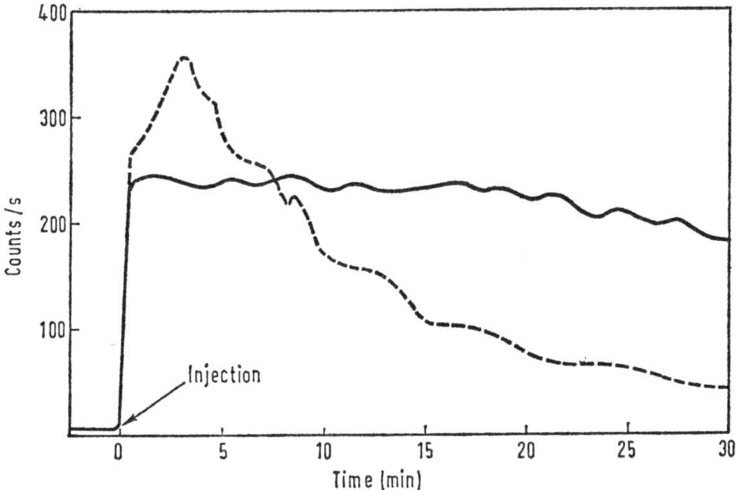

Fig. 27 Renogram revealing defective left kidney. Broken line, right kidney (normal). Full line, left kidney.

Renography

The kidneys have two important functions. They act as filters, purifying the blood by the removal of waste products and excess salts, and they control the water content of the body by passing excess to the bladder. Their function is therefore essentially mechanical and can be tested by relatively straightforward methods using radio-active tracers. Other tests are available but are difficult, and can involve urethral catheterization and complex chemical procedures.

Using the simple test, a substance such as hippuran (which is readily filtered by the kidneys) is labelled with ^{131}I and injected

D

into the blood-stream. The accumulation and clearance of the tracer is then monitored for 30 min or so with external detectors placed over the kidneys. Often a third detector over the heart monitors the clearance from the blood. The record of such a kidney test is called a renogram. Clearly the slope of the renogram at any time will be a function of the two competing processes, (*a*) the rate of removal of hippuran from the blood to the kidney, and (*b*) the rate of removal from kidney to bladder. Renograms of a patient with a normal right and defective left kidney are shown in fig. 27.

Tracer

In the test just described ^{131}I is the tracer, but other isotopes can also be used. They must be gamma-emitters and the energies of their radiations must be high enough to ensure that there is insignificant absorption in the tissues of the body—otherwise a deeply situated normal kidney could give the same result as one with reduced uptake.

Collimation

Another very important consideration is collimation. Clearly it is essential to restrict the field of view of the detector—a sodium iodide crystal coupled to a photomultiplier tube—so that it can respond to radiation arising only within a well-defined region. However, differences of opinion exist as to the optimum degree of collimation.

One technique is to view the whole kidney with a shielded detector far enough away (25 cm) to ensure that the effect of variations in the kidney-skin distance is small. Here large crystals (7·5 cm diameter × 5 cm thick) compensate for the increased source-detector distance. One difficulty is that it is virtually impossible to allow for variations in the size of the kidney. Other workers have also used 'broad' collimation but have placed the detectors much closer to the body, thereby obviating the need for large crystals but making the results highly sensitive to the kidney-skin distances.

The second technique is 'narrow' collimation. Here the lead shield which defines the field of view of the crystal may be in the form of a long narrow cylinder, possibly 15 cm long and 2·5 cm in internal diameter. Providing that the wall of the cylinder is thick enough (1·0 to 2·0 cm) to reduce to a negligible level the possibility that radiation may penetrate the collimator, the field of view can be approximately determined from simple optical considerations, and at the kidneys will be some 3·7 to 5·0 cm wide.

The 'sensitive' volume of the kidney will then be roughly cylindrical in shape and the variation from kidney to kidney will be in thickness only (as against volume with broad collimation). Within reason, the detector-skin distance is not critical as the count rate is independent of distance, providing that the object fills the whole field of view of the detector.

Equipment

Data from tests are collected and processed in a relatively straight-forward manner. The output from each of the two, or possibly three, sodium iodide crystal-photomultiplier assemblies is amplified with a gain of approximately a hundred and filtered through a pulse-height selector which will reject most of the noise and discriminate against scattered radiation. The filtered pulses drive a ratemeter which can generally accommodate frequencies from 3 to 3000 counts/s in seven or eight ranges; 200 counts/s is a typical maximum rate during the test.

The ratemeter outputs are normally displayed on a multi-pen potentiometric recorder with chart speed of approximately 50 cm/h. There is probably something to be said for using a greater chart speed during the first two or three minutes of the test as some information can be obtained from a detailed study of early uptakes. The stability and reliability of the instruments are of paramount importance as the test will generally be carried out by a person of limited technical ability.

Thyroid function

Iodine is an essential constituent of a hormone, excreted by the thyroid gland, that controls body metabolism. When disease of the thyroid is suspected valuable information can be obtained by studying the rate of accumulation in the gland of trace amounts of radio-active iodine. The test is straightforward. A small dose (approximately 5 μCi) of ^{131}I is given orally and at certain times thereafter the count rate due to the isotope in the gland (as measured by a collimated sodium iodide scintillation detector about 20 cm from the neck) is compared with the count rate due to the same dose in a neck phantom. Comparisons are made at selected times during the first two days of the test.

In this test the activity in the gland remains constant throughout each counting period (e.g. 1 min) and a scaler is used in preference to a ratemeter. In some specialized investigations of thyroid function the rate of accumulation in the first few minutes after injection is studied, and a ratemeter coupled to a potentiometric recorder is more suitable.

Lung function

Oxygenation of blood occurs through thin membranes that separate the tiny air sacs from the small blood vessels in the lungs. The efficiency of exchange in a region of the lung depends on the amount of air reaching the region (ventilation) and the amount of blood flowing through the region (perfusion). Both ventilation and perfusion can be studied using radio-active inert gases and external scintillation counters.

In a study of ventilation the patient inhales air containing radio-active ^{133}Xe. The distribution of the xenon can then be studied using either of two techniques. In the first a number (usually six) of regions of the chest are viewed using a stationary array of collimated sodium iodide crystal detectors. In the second, a pair of detectors scans the chest rapidly (in 10 s) from top to bottom. In both cases the signals from the detectors are amplified, analysed and fed into ratemeters. The analogue outputs from the ratemeters are displayed on multi-channel potentiometric recorders.

Perfusion can be studied by injecting radio-active ^{133}Xe dissolved in saline into a vein and studying the accumulation of xenon in the lungs by either of the above methods.

There are other tests that involve the same kind of equipment as that described above. In some of the tests several detectors are used to monitor the activities in various regions. One complication is that, if the test is very short (of the order of minutes), the settings on the various instruments (i.e. ranges in the ratemeters) cannot be optimized in the time. In these circumstances it is advisable to take down the data on a multi-channel tape recorder and analyse the results later.

Thermography

Considerable interest has been aroused recently by developments in the relatively new field of thermography, the diagnosis of disease by infra-red detection methods. The precision is remarkably good. With one of the more advanced instruments in the field the exposed body or part of the body is scanned some sixteen times a second, using a remote infra-red detector, and the temperature patterns of the skin are displayed on an oscilloscope. Temperature abnormalities of as little as 0·2°C can be readily detected.

Applied clinically the technique is painless, safe and non-destructive, and is used in conditions where disease produces abnormal skin temperature patterns owing to increased metabolism or to local circulatory disturbances. In breast cancer a marked temperature difference has been reported, ranging from 1 to 5°C, between the skin over the affected site and the skin over the normal breast. Moreover, the magnitude of the difference can often indicate the likelihood of secondary cancers.

Other fields in which thermography is being used with increasing success include the painless assessment of skin burns, the investigation of circulatory disturbances, studies of rheumatoid arthritis and placental location.

Physics of thermography

It is well known that a surface at a temperature above absolute zero loses energy by thermal radiation and that the spectrum of the electromagnetic radiation depends on the temperature and nature of the surface. In this context the behaviour of human skin at normal ambient temperatures is virtually identical with that of a dull black body.

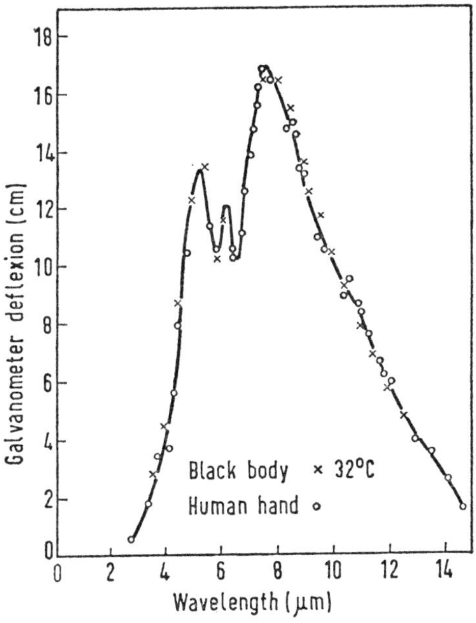

Fig. 28 Spectrum of black body emission at 32°C compared with human hand emission at similar temperatures. (After Hardy, *Physics in Medicine and Biology*, 1934, Vol. 9, No. 4, p. 435.) (*Courtesy of Taylor and Francis Ltd.*)

At 32°C the radiation has a spectrum of wavelengths lying in a broad peak essentially between 2 μm and 15 μm, with a maximum at about 8 μm (fig. 28). This is in good agreement with Planck's law, which applies only to black body radiation. The wavelength, λ_{max}, at which maximal emission occurs is a function of the temperature of the surface. By Wien's displacement law $\lambda_{max.} = 2880/T$, where λ is the wavelength in micrometres and T the surface temperature in degrees Kelvin.

It is evident from these laws that there will be little variation in the shape of the emission spectrum within the range of normal skin temperatures, so the infra-red detector need only have a response between 2 and 15 μm.

Detectors

Two types of detector are used in thermal-scanning devices.

First there are the temperature-sensitive systems, such as thermistors, which respond to a wide band of the spectrum but are comparatively slow in response because of their finite thermal capacities. A successful commercial scanner has been built using this type of detector.

Second there are the thermosensitive detectors, such as the indium antimonide photoconductive cell. This has an extremely rapid response, of the order of a few microseconds, but under normal operating conditions responds only to radiation within the band from visible to 5·5 μm and therefore only to a small fraction of the emission spectrum from the naked skin. Refrigeration is necessary to reduce noise; normally liquid nitrogen (−190°C) is used as the refrigerant. In clinical applications the mismatch between the waveband of optimum response and the waveband of maximum emission reduces the sensitivity of the device but enhances the temperature contrast because the variation of emitted power with body-surface temperature is large in the overlapping band.

Instruments

A.G.A. (Sweden) have developed a device (Thermovision) which is essentially a thermal television system presenting the temperature distribution of an object as a picture on an oscilloscope screen. The operation is similar to that of a closed-circuit television system with camera and display unit.

A schematic diagram of the Thermovision Model 652 is shown in fig. 29. Incoming infra-red radiation is focused (using the spherical mirror) on to a plane mirror which oscillates at 16 Hz about a horizontal axis, thereby scanning the field of view vertically. A four-sided prism, turning about a vertical axis at 400 rev/s, effectively scans the frame horizontally. The arrangements are equivalent to a 100-line television system with a frame rate of 16 frames/s.

The field of view is a function of the focal distance, being some 15 cm wide by 18 cm high at the minimum local distance of 2 m. The limit of optical resolution is about 3 mm at 2 m. Temperature discrimination of better than 0·5°C is possible by visual observation of the cathode-ray screen. This can be improved to about 0·2°C by using a cathode-ray tube with a long-persistence phosphor. The detector, an indium antimonide cell cooled by liquid nitrogen, responds to radiation within the band 2·0 to 5·4 μm, the upper limit

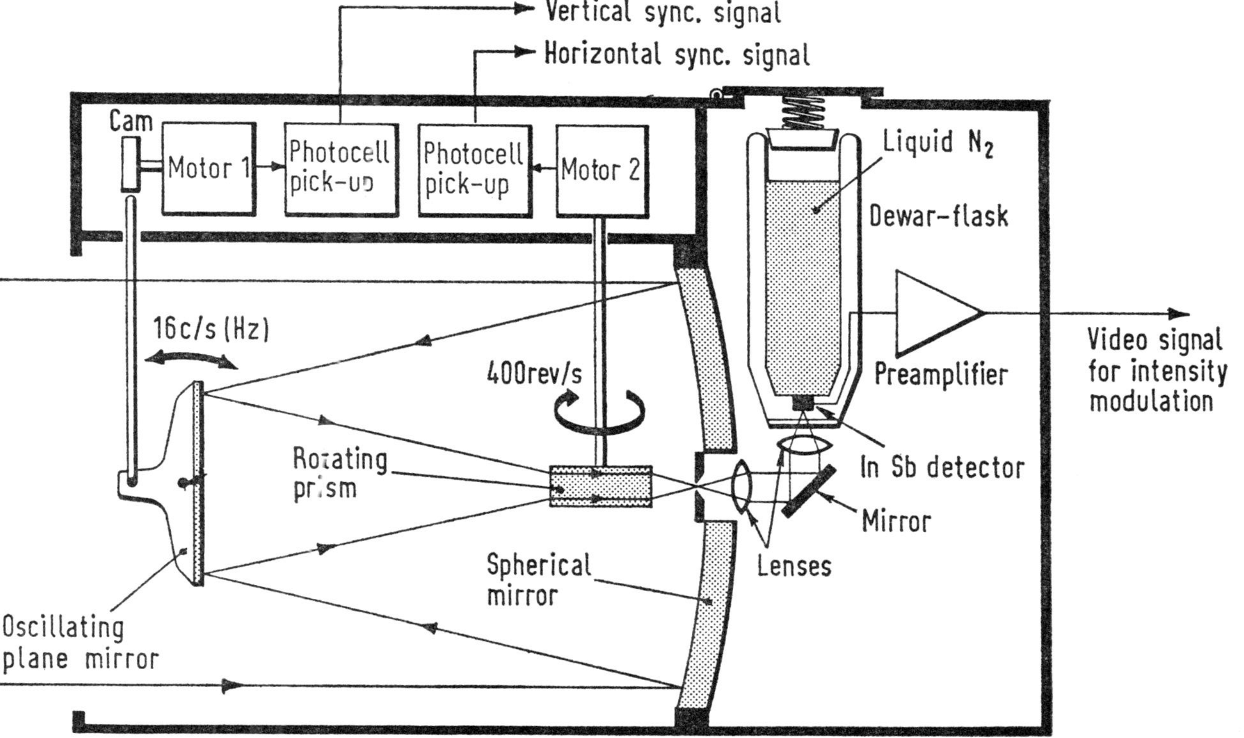

Fig. 29 Schematic diagram of A.G.A. Thermovision model 652 thermal television system.

being set by the detector and the lower limit by the optical properties.

Using brightness and contrast controls one can select the appropriate temperature level and temperature range. Calibration is possible with a reference scale which is continuously displayed on the screen. A wide temperature band is available but is not essential for clinical applications.

Smiths Medical Equipment also market an instrument which uses an indium antimonide detector. Optical and temperature resolution are good but the method of data presentation differs from that of the Swedish instrument and scanning is slower, some 30s being required for one picture.

Future trends

At the moment the field is in the state—often met in medicine—in which the precision of the instruments exceeds the requirements demanded clinically. This situation may not last long after extensive clinical trials and evaluation of the potential of the method. Thought could be given, however, to development of an instrument which gives a well-defined, life-size picture of the scanned region—possibly by using more lines on the television system.

Ultrasonics

Ultrasonics, the science of mechanical vibration at frequencies above the limit of audibility (about 20 kHz) has been increasingly used in medicine over the past decade. Therapeutic applications are few and are not relevant to this chapter. But considerable diagnostic use has been made of a simple pulse-echo principle in many fields, including neurosurgery, ophthalmology, obstetrics, gynaecology and cardiology. A beam of ultrasonic pulses, externally generated, is transmitted into an organ and the pattern of echoes from internal discontinuities is displayed on an oscilloscope screen. Often the same probe acts both as transmitter and receiver. Various other techniques have been used and the range of available instruments is expanding rapidly.

Frequency

The optimum operating frequency is strongly influenced by two factors, resolution and absorption. For maximum spatial resolution a high frequency is required. The velocity of sound in the body depends on the type of tissue but is generally close to the velocity in water (1500 m/s). At 1 MHz the wavelength is approximately 1·5 mm, which gives an indication of the spatial resolution at this frequency.

However, absorption, which is exponential, is approximately proportional to frequency. The thickness for 50 per cent reduction in sound pressure in most of the tissues of the body is of the order of 5 to 10 cm at 1 MHz. In bone, the half-thickness is down by a factor of approximately ten. In every application, therefore, a compromise has to be made.

In practice, 6 MHz (wavelength 0·25 mm) is about optimum for studies of the eye although frequencies up to 15 MHz can be used when only the front of the eye is being examined. A lower frequency has to be used in investigations of the deeper organs such as the brain, where absorption in the skull is high and where probably 1 to 2 MHz is best.

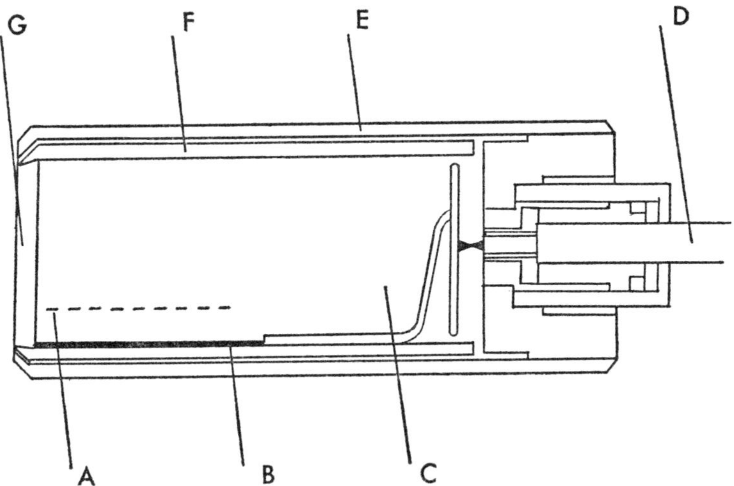

Fig. 30 A typical contact-type ultrasonic probe

    A = Earth connexions to transducer
    B = Line connexion to transducer
    C = Tungsten-araldite mixture as 'backing block'
    D = Cable
    E = Outer case
    F = Inner case
    G = Transducer disc of barium titanate or lead zirconate/titanate

Generation

Ultrasound can be generated by the magnetostrictive effect in ferromagnetic materials, by the piezo-electric effect in most crystals lacking centres of symmetry, and by an effect akin to the piezo-electric effect in certain specially treated ceramics. Under normal conditions, the upper frequency limit by the first is about 100 kHz, which is not high enough for optimum clinical use. In the normal mode of operation, that of thickness resonance, the maximum practical frequency using piezo-electric crystals and ceramics is of the order of hundreds of megahertz, which is quite adequate for medical applications. To date, microwave ultrasonics have found no application in the medical field.

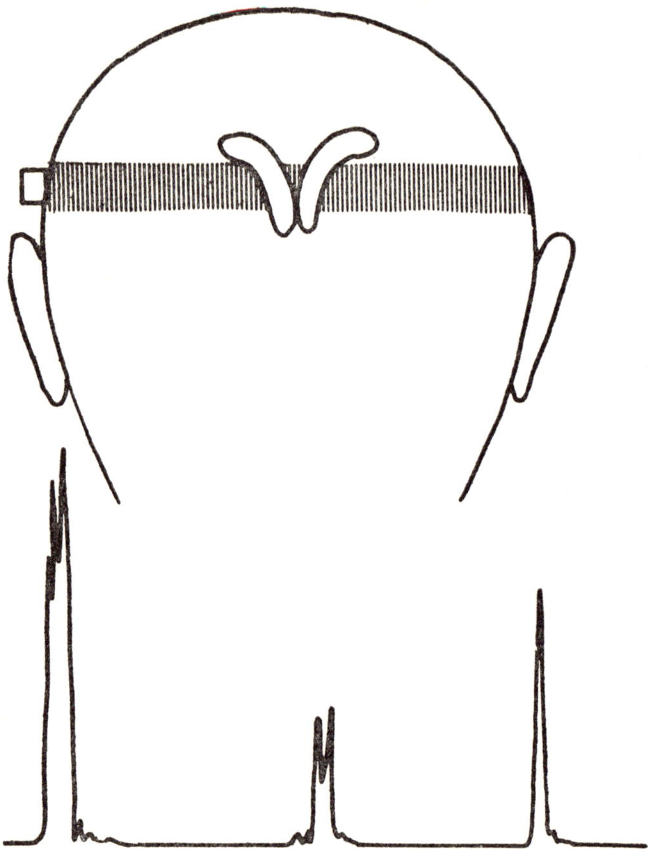

Fig. 31 A-scanning of head. Normal A-scan shows echoes from the mid-line and the skull. (T. G. Brown, *Ultrasonics*, April 1967.) (*Courtesy of Iliffe Publications Ltd.*)

Transducers

Normally the transducers used clinically are in the form of disks or plates half a wavelength thick (fig. 30). From these the intensity is proportional both to the square of the exciting voltage (V) and the square of the piezo-electric stress constant (e). In piezo-electric crystals, e.g. of quartz, e is less by a factor of about a hundred than in ceramics, e.g. barium titanate and lead zirconate. To achieve the same intensity, V has to be greater by the same factor. Ceramic transducers are normally used when high power is required, but quartz is suitable for diagnosis.

Air gaps between the transducers and the body have to be avoided as they reflect most of the energy of the ultrasonic beams. Good sonic contact can be achieved using a coupling fluid such as a mineral oil.

Measurement

The total power in an ultrasonic beam can be monitored either calorimetrically or by radiation pressure measurements. In the calorimetric approach the temperature increase due to the absorption of ultrasound in a chamber of liquid (generally water) is compared with the increase due to electrical heating. In the second approach the radiation pressure due to the reflexion of ultrasound at an interface is measured by means of a simple pressure balance immersed in water. The results agree to within 10 per cent.

The intensity distribution can be studied using a tiny thermo-couple probe immersed in a small chamber filled with a strongly absorbing liquid like castor oil. Intensities down to 1 W/cm^2 at 1 MHz can be detected. In a transparent medium the diffraction of light in an ultrasonic beam can be calibrated to give intensity distribution.

Mode of operation

In the simplest instruments that use the pulse-echo technique the signals received when ultrasonic pulses are reflected from internal discontinuities in the body organ are displayed as ordinates on a cathode ray oscilloscope. In this mode (A-scope) a one-dimensional picture of the reflecting interface is shown (fig. 31). Frequencies within the range 1 to 15 MHz are used and each pulse lasts several microseconds. Repetition rates between 100 and 1000 pulses/s are required. The amplitudes of the reflected signals do not yield much useful information and in some instruments the range of amplitudes of the signals displayed is compressed (using, for example, amplifiers with logarithmic responses). Generally the echoes from discontinuities deep in the organ are of low amplitude. They can be compensated for in other instruments by using amplifiers with gains controlled by the pulse-echo intervals.

A more sophisticated technique (B-scanning) can, however, give a two-dimensional picture of the interface pattern (fig. 32). The organ is scanned with a probe that moves over the organ at right-angles to the direction of the beam. The pattern is displayed on an oscilloscope; the X-deflexion of the spot indicates the position of the probe and the Y-deflexion the pulse-echo interval.

One disadvantage of these techniques is that only those discontinuities that are approximately normal to the direction of the beam give

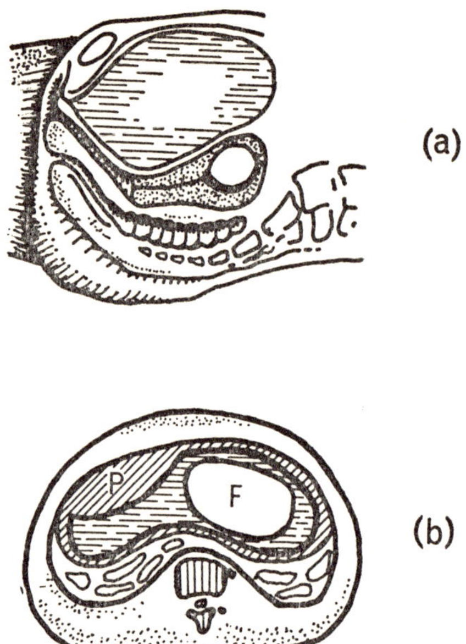

Fig. 32 Image of womb showing (*a*) 6-week gestation sac behind full bladder and (*b*) transverse cross-section with placenta (P) and foetal trunk (F) at 28 weeks. (*After photographs by courtesy of Dept. of Ultrasonic Technology, Glasgow University.*)

detectable echoes. The limitations so imposed can be overcome by various techniques, such as radial scanning, sector scanning, compound sector scanning and compound B-scanning (fig. 33). In radial scanning the detector surveys the organ in an arc so that the beam is transmitted into the body at various angles. In sector scanning the detector, which is in direct contact with a fixed point on the surface of the body, is rotated to vary the direction of the beam. Compound sector scanning is sector scanning from a large number of points on the surface of the body. In compound B-scanning, B-scans of limited width are carried out over a number of regions.

Ultrasonic image camera

All these techniques rely on the pulse-echo principle, but one instrument that operates on an entirely different principle is the ultrasonic image camera. This instrument, which was developed to detect flaws in materials, has not yet been used to any extent in medicine but has considerable clinical potential. A continuous beam of ultrasound is generated by a transmitter approximately 50 cm from the object. The transmitted beam falls on a plate of piezo-electric material (quartz or

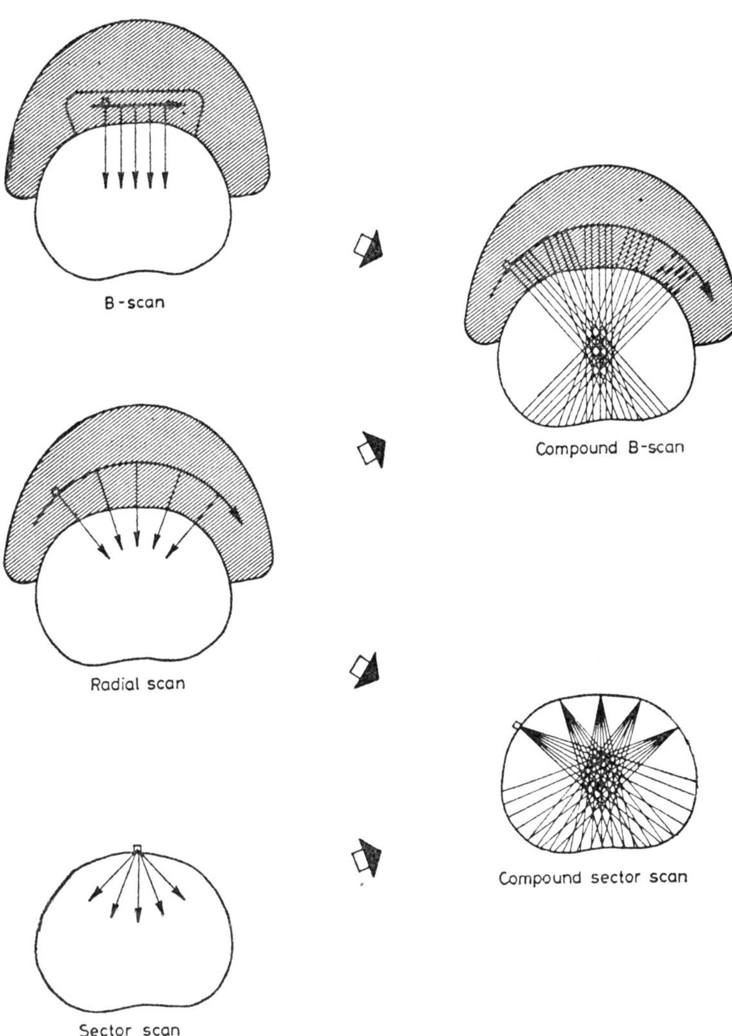

Fig. 33 Simple scanning techniques (*left*) are combined in compound scanning (*right*). Shaded areas represent water-coupling baths. (T. G. Brown, *Ultrasonics,* April 1967.) (*Courtesy of Iliffe Publications Ltd.*)

barium titanate) producing at each point a voltage that is proportional to the incident energy. The back of the plate is scanned many times each second by a beam from an electron gun, and the current of secondary electrons produced (which is proportional to the voltage at each point) is amplified by an electron multiplier. The amplified signal goes to an oscilloscope screen which is being scanned in synchronism. In this way the pattern of interface is displayed on the screen.

Instruments based on Doppler effect

Another interesting development in ultrasonics in recent years has been the introduction of techniques that use the Doppler effect to identify moving and pulsating objects. When sound is reflected from a moving surface the frequency of the echo is either increased or decreased, depending upon whether the surface is moving towards or away from the source. Interference between ultrasound reflected from stationary surfaces and ultrasound, of a slightly different frequency, reflected from a moving surface causes beats of a frequency dependent on the velocity of the moving surface. The beats are detected and processed electronically to produce audible signals.

Instruments based on this technique are being increasingly applied in gynaecology, cardiology and neurology. In particular, for example, foetal heart beats can be detected at an earlier stage in pregnancy, using one of these instruments, than by conventional techniques (such as foetal electrocardiography).

Future developments

Developments in ultrasonics appear to be following roughly the same pattern as in radio-isotope scanning, and it is possible that ultrasonic image cameras or developments from them will eventually replace the more simple, conventional instruments.

CHAPTER 6

BEDSIDE AND BENCH

In a book on medical instrumentation, written by physicists, it is understandable that pride of place is given to the measurement of physical quantities such as temperature, pressure and flow rate by the direct use of instruments working on physical principles and depending on the technology derived from them. But the science which is most frequently and most directly applied to the investigation of illness and to the control of therapeutic procedures is biochemistry. From a few simple tests conducted with test tubes over spirit lamps in ward side-rooms, through the stage of being an appendage of the pathology department, biochemical science and technology has led to the development of busy departments of clinical chemistry with a vital role in the hospital service.

For years these medical laboratories have been faced with an ever-growing demand for an increasing variety of measurements. Fig. 34

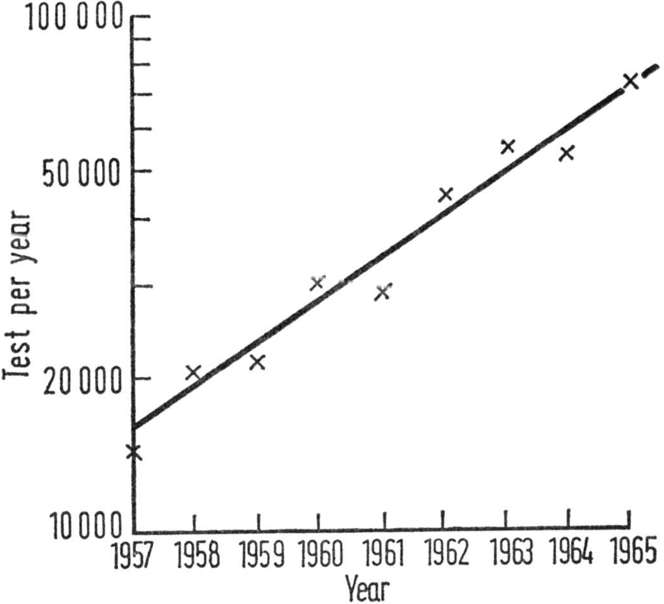

Fig. 34 Numbers of routine tests done in the clinical chemistry laboratories of a Scottish teaching hospital with 550 beds.

shows the increase in work load of a medium-sized teaching hospital in Scotland over a period of nine years: the work load increases at a rate of 20 per cent per annum. Figures from other hospitals show very similar rates of growth, with doubling times of four years.

In the early stages of this development the techniques involved the use of much staff time and some primitive, cheap items of equipment. Burettes, pipettes and other items familiar to us in our school days were the standard tools: the sight of a substantial piece of equipment indicated a research project supported by a special grant. Although many changes have taken place, the heritage of the past still lingers and impedes progress.

The only hope of bringing to the patient the technology which modern science supports, of keeping pace with the explosive dis-coveries of the biochemist, lies in the maximum application of instru-ment technology in the laboratory. This transition brings many problems to the hospital service. The need for continuing large capital investment in equipment is difficult to meet. The hospital service—in Britain and other countries—is still mainly geared to paying large bills to maintain premises and staff while providing only trivial equipment—scalpels, stethoscopes and the like. Laboratory accommodation is almost always severely inadequate. Even a new building is generally too small by the date of occupation, for few planning authorities can be made to believe that the work load will continue to rise exponentially. There are problems in adapting the staffing structure, which was devised to provide labour for a large load of simple operations.

The need for maintenance and repair of technical equipment is new to the hospital service—the expenditure on maintenance services at present is astonishingly small, covering mainly heating, lighting, plumbing and carpentry. It is still possible for an authority to pur-chase complex analytical equipment costing £20000 and include only a £20 multi-range meter and a few hand tools for calibration, checking, maintenance and repair.

Although these difficulties make progress uneven, there is no doubt that equipment now tried and tested in the advanced laboratories will become standard in all hospital laboratories in a few years. In the following pages it is not possible to do more than outline some of the more important or more novel instruments.

Spectrometry

Spectroscopy—the identification and assay of a substance by recording the spectrum of emitted light after electrons are raised to higher energy levels—is one of the well-established techniques. From the visually-observed flame test to the simple flame photometer with transmission light filters and photocell is a small step, but one which gives good results in measuring the alkali metals in solution. The use of several filters and photomultipliers allows simultaneous determinations of several elements, usually with one used as an internal standard.

When there is interference from other elements in the sample—magnesium often causes trouble—a monochromator is preferable to filters. It is then normal to use the burner in conjunction with a general-purpose spectrophotometer which can also be employed to investigate spectra in the visible and ultra-violet.

The spectrophotometer consists of a light source, a monochromator to select a narrow waveband, a transparent cell containing a solution of the sample to be investigated and a light detector to measure the intensity of light transmitted by the cell. The intensity is compared with that of the light passing through an identical reference cell containing solvent but no sample.

There is a high degree of sophistication in modern equipment. An example is the Unicam SP700 recording spectrophotometer. Either a prism monochromator or a diffraction grating may be used; with a grating the dispersion is more nearly constant throughout the spectrum. Sensitive photomultipliers are employed, and the currents are amplified by a.c. amplifiers tuned to the frequency at which the light is mechanically chopped. Rather than carry out serial measurements on sample and reference cell, one can have a split beam and the ratio indicated immediately. An absorption spectrum is required more often than an absorption measurement at a single wavelength, and the scanning mechanism of the monochromator and chart recorder are linked to give a fully automatic system.

Further efforts to improve the already high sensitivity and reliability of such instruments seem likely to bring diminishing returns in clinical practice, but continued improvement in the ease of analysis of very small sample volumes would be welcome in many applications.

Many organic substances show characteristic fluorescence when irradiated with ultra-violet light, and spectrofluorimeters are among the most useful instruments in the laboratory. They are often simple instruments with mercury vapour lamps, quartz cells for liquid samples, a selection of interference filters or liquid filter cells and photomultiplier detectors.

Several metals are estimated by spraying a liquid sample into a flame and measuring the emission or absorption of light which is characteristic of the element. Since there are more atoms in the ground state than in the higher states the absorption method is more sensitive than the flame emission. It is also less affected by interference from other elements present. The light source is a hollow-cathode lamp of the metal to be determined.

The possibility of extending the lower wavelength limit to include the far ultra-violet region, in which lie the electronic absorption levels of many molecules, is not promising. Interest turns to the infra-red region, in which most molecules show rotation and vibration absorption. The infra-red spectra are so complex that dealing with mixtures of compounds is scarcely practicable. The technique is most useful in identifying a complex molecule and studying its structure, since some groups of atoms have characteristic absorption wavelengths relatively unaffected by the remainder of the molecule. Fully automatic machines are required: the double-beam design is most common, with an electronic null point produced by an optical attenuator driven by a servo-motor.

In the Hilger and Watts Infrascan recording infra-red spectrophotometer, solid samples may be mixed with potassium bromide powder and compressed to form a transparent disk. A special, simple application of infra-red absorption is found in apparatus for estimation of respiratory gases and anaesthetic gases and vapours.

In optically active substances the variation with wavelength of the rotation of the plane of polarization of light gives a sensitive method of investigation, mainly used in research at present. Powerful light sources and sensitive detectors are essential: in simple polarimeters the end-point occurs when polarizer and analyser are crossed and extinction is complete. For greater sensitivity the beam is split into two parts before the analyser, the direction of polarization being rotated slightly in opposite senses for the two beams. The final position of the analyser results in equal intensity in the two halves, rather than complete extinction. As in other applications of spectrophotometry, extension further into the ultra-violet is desirable.

In principle, X-ray spectra do not differ from spectra of visible or ultra-violet light produced by electronic energy changes, but the instrumental requirements for recording them are quite different. X-ray techniques are applicable only to elemental analysis and may be used for all elements except those of very low atomic numbers. Below sodium, the detection of the long-wave radiation becomes too difficult for routine practice.

There are two methods of exciting the atoms. Most commonly the sample is irradiated with X-rays from a conventional X-ray tube operating between 10 and 100 keV, the higher values being needed only if elements of high atomic number are to be detected. The photoelectric absorption in the specimen is followed by the emission of characteristic or fluorescent X-rays—the K, L, etc., lines.

The less common method of excitation is to make a solid specimen the target of the X-ray tube, bombarding it with a beam of electrons. If a micro-beam is made to scan the specimen the distribution of the element across the specimen may be examined in fine detail. At present this is an exciting research tool.

The X-radiation from excited atoms is analysed by an X-ray spectrometer—collimator, crystal and detector. The crystal is rotated so that the wavelength which is characteristic of the element of interest reaches the detector—usually a scintillation counter, or, for longer-wave radiation, a proportional counter. The count rate is measured by standard nucleonic apparatus and is proportional to the mass of the element, provided that absorption by other elements is allowed for. Simultaneous and quite automatic analysis for several specified elements is possible. Alternatively, a complete spectrum of a sample with unknown constituents can be recorded. Fig. 35 shows an X-ray spectrum of a specimen containing lines of six elements.

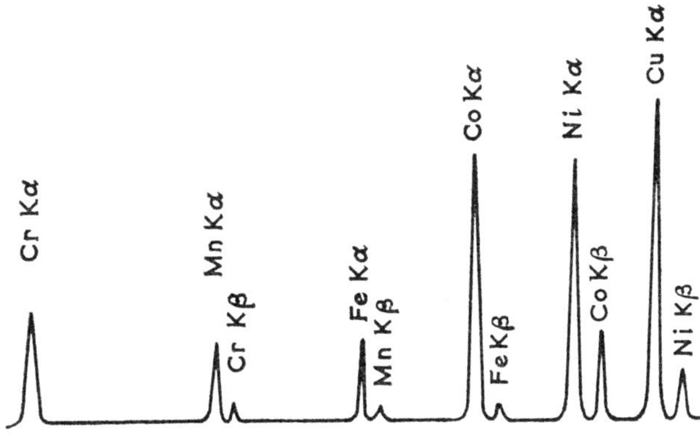

Fig. 35 An X-ray fluorescent spectrum.

Perhaps because the potential user is not introduced to expensive modern equipment through relatively simple versions (as in the case of optical spectrometry) the technique is as yet rarely used. For a few elements its sensitivity is better than that of optical methods; for many it could become quicker.

Activation analysis

Activation analysis is a powerful modern technique for quantitative elemental analysis. The sample is exposed to neutrons to form radio-isotopes of elements present, and the wanted element is determined by radio-active assay techniques.

One approach is to use simple nucleonic counting equipment and rely on standard chemical techniques to separate the wanted element from others in the sample. In addition to the inherently high sensitivity of radio-isotope assay procedures, this has the advantage over a simple chemical analysis that, after activation, the reagents need not be free from the element sought—indeed, large amounts may be added as a carrier—since only the activated atoms in the original sample can be detected.

An approach more interesting to the instrument technologist—though less practicable for most laboratories—is to separate the elements present by disentangling the characteristic gamma-ray spectra. Given sufficient investment the analytical system can be made fully automatic.

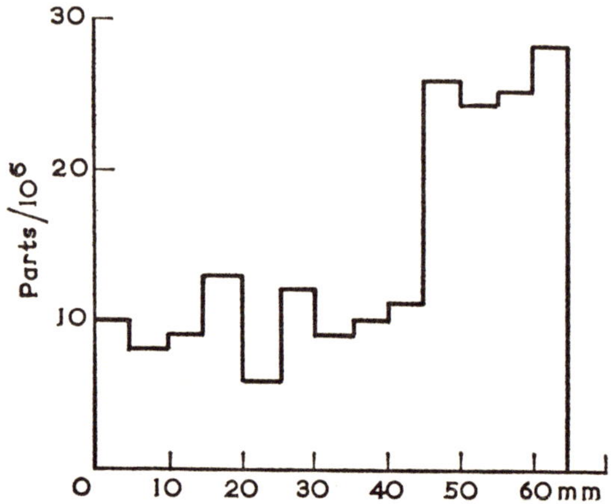

Fig. 36 Example of activation analysis for arsenic, showing distribution along hair of patient with arsenical poisoning.

Activation analysis has been applied to problems in forensic science and industrial health, where poisonous trace elements are important, and to research on the role of trace elements in the body. Fig. 36 shows the distribution of arsenic along the length of a single hair taken from a patient with arsenical poisoning.

The usefulness of activation analysis varies for the elements, depending on their neutron-capture cross-section* and on the characteristics of the radio-isotope produced. One trace element with an important biological function is iodine, and body levels of this element present a difficult analytical problem. A successful iodine activation technique has been developed in one laboratory (it has been sought by several groups of workers), and will undoubtedly become widely used.

Activation analysts have generally relied on nuclear reactors as neutron sources. For many elements the most sensitive techniques are based on activation with thermal neutrons, as given by a reactor. Compact generators now available at modest cost (under £10000

* The neutron-capture cross-section of an atomic nucleus is a measure of the probability of capture of a neutron by that nucleus.

with counting equipment and other accessories) give useful outputs of fast neutrons, which serve for activation of several light elements (atomic number less than 10) and may be used in special circumstances for work with heavier elements. Fast neutron activation analysis is generally less sensitive but is more convenient for on-line estimation and process control.

Electrochemical methods

Several varied electrochemical techniques are used in clinical chemistry. The most important is probably pH measurement, and the pH meter employing a glass electrode is commonplace. A sensitive, linear, d.c. amplifier with high input-impedance is essential, and all standard systems, from direct coupling to chopper amplifiers, are used. Earlier workers found difficulty in obtaining reliable and stable electrodes, but the difficulties are less troublesome today. On a similar basis is the measurement of the partial pressure of carbon dioxide and the bicarbonate concentration.

Polarography with a dropping-mercury electrode has not been used in biochemical laboratories as extensively as in industry. As well as trace metals and inorganic ions, some organic compounds can be reduced at a mercury cathode and measured by obtaining the current–voltage curve for small currents flowing to the fresh surface of the small, forming, mercury drop. Compounds which are normally inert can sometimes be converted into a form which can be determined polarographically. Closely related molecules can be analysed in a mixture, and the procedure is suitable for micro-assay. Apparatus is available for rapid, automatic recording of the polarographic waveform and its first derivative.

Electrodes other than the mercury drop may be used for special purposes. The partial pressure of oxygen in blood can be so measured. The cathode is of platinum or gold. The anode is of silver in potassium chloride, or in a similar conducting gel contained in a semi-permeable membrane through which the oxygen diffuses.

Chromatography, electrophoresis and other physical separation techniques

Identification and assay of the components of a mixture is greatly assisted by chromatography, electrophoresis and similar techniques by which components can be spatially separated owing to physical differences such as differences in partition coefficient or in particle charge, size and shape.

The earliest, and perhaps the simplest, methods of identifying the separated components involved chemical reactions leading to visible colour changes. They gave rise to the name *chromatography*, which is not now descriptive of the technique's many developments. Other, often more sophisticated, methods of quantitative and qualitative analysis are now applied to the fractions.

All methods of chromatography essentially rely on the distribution of a sample between a stationary and a moving phase.

In the first and most common method the moving phase is a liquid. The stationary phase may be a finely divided absorbing solid, an ion-exchange resin, a molecular sieve or a liquid supported on a solid. The stationary-phase material may be packed in a column. Alternatively, the absorbing material may be in the form of a thin layer. Paper, the most commonly used material, is a special case of the thin-layer system.

According to the relative rates of diffusion and interchange between moving and stationary phases, components of a mixture introduced at the inflow will travel through at different rates. Ideally, the components will be spatially separated in the system: a thin layer of paper can be scanned by a detector—particularly useful where radio-isotope labelling is used—or cut up into fractions. At the exit point the components emerge at different times, and the effluent can be analysed continuously by an instrument, e.g. spectrophotometrically, spectrofluorometrically, or by scintillation counting in tubes made of plastic phosphor. Alternatively, discrete samples can be automatically collected at the exit. Where only one component is wanted it may be possible to add a radio-active substance which travels slightly faster and energizes the collecting system.

Even greater versatility and sensitivity is achieved when the moving phase is a gas into which the sample is introduced in vaporized form. The advantages are gained at the expense of elaboration in the injection and collection systems and in control of parameters such as temperature.

A high degree of separation of components in complex biological mixtures can be achieved. Fig. 37 shows the separation of some steroids by gas–liquid chromatography.

Efficient detection of the separated components presents an interesting challenge. The commonly used detectors are based on changes in thermal conductivity or density of the gas, or changes in electrical conductivity after ionization by a flame or a radio-active source. Mass spectrometry is very suitable for the identification of small quantities of isolated gaseous compounds. Combined with gas chromatography it is a powerful, if very expensive, analytical technique. It can be expected to develop in the directions of simplification and specialization. Gas chromatography is obviously readily applicable to the analysis of gases in blood or to respiratory gas samples, and special equipment is available for these purposes.

In electrophoresis the separation occurs when charged particles of the mixture move under the influence of an electric field through a liquid held in a supporting medium. Complete separation of components occurs in zone electrophoresis, the most common form. Paper has been widely used as a supporting medium but the advantages of polyacrylamide gels have recently become evident. Detection and quantitative assay techniques are similar to those used in thin-layer chromatography, with spectrophotometry as the most popular instrumental method.

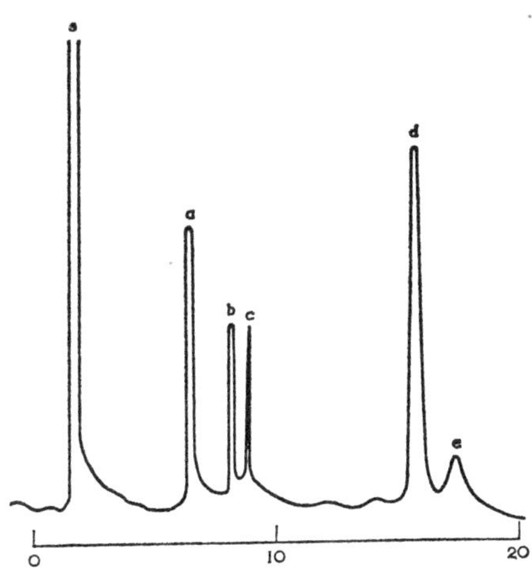

Fig. 37 Steroid separation by gas–liquid chromatography.

s = solvent   a = pregnenolone
b = progesterone   c = squalene
d = cholesterol   e = $\triangle^7$ cholesterol

Electrophoresis is an excellent method of separating proteins, nucleic acids and other significant constituents in clinical samples. With relatively simple apparatus small specimens can be handled. Many good power supplies are now marketed, giving choice of constant-voltage or constant-current operation, and tanks giving adequate control of parameters need no longer be improvised or constructed by the user.

Many other physical instruments and techniques find application in some specialized assay or in biochemical research. Paramagnetic properties of oxygen are used in oxygen analysis. Electron spin resonance and nuclear magnetic resonance are valuable in some research fields. A progressive laboratory uses radio-isotope techniques extensively to improve standard clinical methods.

The future

Looking to the future one may predict two trends.

Although further sophisticated tests can be expected, the most welcomed developments in the near future will be those which permit automatic performance of a number of tests on one small sample. The first such instrument, the Technicon Auto-analyser, revolutionized much of the routine in clinical chemistry. Its value lay in the ingenuity with which it automated relatively orthodox methods of analysis, mainly ending in colorimetric estimation. Equal ingenuity applied to other, perhaps physically more elaborate, procedures is to be expected.

In the more distant future we may expect more direct application of instrumentation to the intact patient to measure the biochemical parameters *in vivo*, particularly during periods of intensive care. This will call for micro-miniaturization of transducers, and perhaps for internal spectrophotometry using fibre optics. Experiments are in progress on activation analysis *in vivo*.

Extracting information is not the only problem—the information must be readily available and must be used wisely. Continuing development of clinical chemistry laboratories must be accompanied by improvements in clinical data handling and in the use of computer techniques to examine the significance of the greater mass of data available. Education of the user is no less important. Full value will be obtained from the development of technology based on science only if it is accompanied by increased ability to develop scientific concepts.

CHAPTER 7

PROSPECTS AND PITFALLS

The greatest achievement of mankind during the last century has been the conquest of disease.

Of course it is true that there are many parts of the world where the hazards of life have altered little during this time, or where people who used to die of malaria are now dying of starvation. The inhabitants of prosperous countries, who might once have died of fever or other infectious illness are now dying of cancer or heart disease in greater numbers than ever. But in general we are very much healthier than our ancestors.

Science and technology have contributed substantially to this change and the association is by no means finished; but it is declining in effectiveness. The gap between the promise and potentiality of modern technology and its application in the realm of medicine is widening rapidly. This is not the impression that would be gained from the popular organs of opinion and enlightenment, which daily record in enthusiastic terms the latest breakthrough in medical instrumentation; but the spectacular benefits offered on these occasions never seem to materialize.

Why is the gap widening? A simple answer (which is partly correct) is to say that not enough money is being spent on health and the activities that contribute to it. In wealthy countries, such as Britain, health comes next to defence and education in cost to public or private funds. Yet there is a considerable pressure to spend even more. An increase can probably be justified by cold economic arguments if in no other way. Better health means a bigger working population and an increase in the gross national product. The drugs which have reduced the incidence of tuberculosis so sharply during the last twenty years are in this way contributing a benefit of some £60m a year in Britain.

Expenditure on health is, however, not decided on this basis. The neglect of science and technology in the hospital service—or, to put it more mildly, the failure to make full use of the benefits now available from advances in these areas of knowledge—is to some extent a consequence of the general paucity of resources for the development of the service.

But it would be wrong to presume that money alone would make a decisive difference in this matter. There are many signs that we do not at present have the attitude of mind or the organization to make more effective use of the abundant possibilities of science and technology in relation to medicine.

The prevailing enthusiasm for computers in medicine offers an example of the pitfalls that await the adventurer in this direction. Computers can be of substantial help in several areas of clinical science—but only if they are properly used. The popular notion that a computer will solve otherwise intractable problems in the diagnosis of disease is not realistic. On the global scale, the major problems in medicine are not those of diagnosis. The killing afflictions, such as malnutrition, cancer and diseases of the heart, are all too easily diagnosed; the trouble is that we do not know how to cope with them afterwards.

Also unrealistic is the hope that a computer will extract significant results from a badly planned experiment, or will increase the information content of a mass of ill-assorted clinical data. The computer is an arithmetical engine, but it is no substitute for the statistical insight that the investigator needs to frame meaningful questions and to interpret the answers.

Another illuminating example is provided by the problem of the cardiac pacemaker. This device uses only a few simple electronic components in a circuit that a very junior engineer could design. It is in great demand in many prosperous countries, and has, indeed, been available from commercial sources for several years. Yet the use of this instrument is attended by disappointment ranging from inconvenience and discomfort to catastrophe. Leads break (some surgeons now implant duplicate leads, knowing that the spare set will be needed before long), terminals corrode (through electrolytic action), output frequencies vary alarmingly, and a host of other unhappy emergencies frustrate the efforts of the surgeon. It would not be difficult to overcome these troubles, many of which arise from failure (or absence) of communication among the various groups of people concerned—designers, manufacturers and users.

The obvious action in such a situation is to establish, before commercial production begins, a representative working party to prepare specifications, allocate research or development contracts if necessary, review competitive tenders and arrange bulk purchase. The procedures are familiar enough in the defence, communications and space industries, but are virtually unknown for medical instrumentation.

In Britain the health departments of the central government are not adequately provided with staff to deal with the problems. Further down the tree, the scientific and technological effort available to the hospital service is too thinly spread. The 250 or so physicists in the National Health Service are distributed among sixty departments, and many of them are occupied largely with activities derived from radiotherapy. The technological support for this modest scientific effort is almost invisible.

The British hospital service—alone among government departments and other substantial users of scientific manpower—does not employ the experimental officers who, in other areas, form the large and essential link between the research scientists and the skilled craftsmen. Consequently some of the work that should be done by properly qualified technologists is neglected, and some is done inefficiently by scientists or craftsmen.

Hospital engineers in Britain are, in the main, concerned with heating, ventilation and electrical installations. There is no provision for instrument technologists, though modern hospitals contain great quantities of control and measuring equipment in wards, theatres and laboratories; in the new hospitals now being planned the need will be even greater.

This chapter had been chiefly concerned with the situation in the hospital service. University departments, Medical Research Council units and other organizations make valuable contributions to medical research—but the greatest need for reinforcement is in the front line. Scientists and technologists (including a few of the highest calibre) should be encouraged to work in hospitals. They should be adequately supported with staff, equipment and other resources.

The interchange of ideas between science and technology is essential for the success of each—and for the well-being of the service with which they are linked. The combination of imaginative basic research with scrupulous attention to tasks arising from the daily routine of clinics, wards and theatres provides the best basis for the formulation of policy to inspire and guide the future applications of science and technology in the realm of medicine.

The achievements which have been reviewed in this book can be vastly extended in the next decade if the necessary effort is made available. This effort will be small in relation to the nation's total commitment and to the recognizable social and economic benefits that will follow.

INDEX